MCQs in Oral and Maxillofacial Pathology with Explanations for PG Dental Entrance Examinations

MCQs in Oral and Maxillofacial Pathology with Explanations for PG Dental Entrance Examinations

Also for BDS & MDS Professional Examinations

Satish Chandra

Best Teacher Awardee
Ex-Member, Dental Council of India
Ex-Director and Professor
Sardar Patel Institute of Dental and Medical Sciences, Lucknow
Ex-Professor and Head of the Department and Dean
Dental Faculty, UP KG University of Dental Sciences (Formerly, KG Medical College, CSM Medical University and KG Medical University, Lucknow)
Ex-Professor, Dean, Head and Principal
DJ College of Dental Sciences and Research, Modinagar, UP
Ex-Professor, Dean, Head and Principal, Institute of Dental Sciences, Bareilly
Ex-Principal, Professor and Head of the Department, Awadh Institute of Dental Sciences, Lucknow
Paper Setter and Examiner of BDS, MDS and PGME
Examinations in Many Universities
Ex-Member, Dental Council of India

Shaleen Chandra

Professor and Head of the Dept., Saraswati Dental College and Hospital, 233 Tiwariganj, Faizabad Road, Juggour, Lucknow
Ex-Professor and Head of the Dept., Sardar Patel Institute of Dental and Medical Sciences, Lucknow
Ex-Assistant Professor, Rama Dental College and Hospital and Research Centre, Kanpur
Ex-Lecturer, UP KG University of Dental Sciences (Formerly, KG Medical College, CSM Medical University and KG Medical University), Lucknow
Ex-Lecturer, Buddha Institute of Dental Sciences, Kankar Bagh, Patna
Paper Setter and Examiner of BDS, MDS and PGME
Examinations in Many Universities

Girish Chandra

Rajendra Nagar Dental Clinic, Lucknow

JAYPEE BROTHERS
MEDICAL PUBLISHERS (P) LTD
New Delhi

Published by

Jitendar P Vij
Jaypee Brothers Medical Publishers (P) Ltd
B-3 EMCA House, 23/23B Ansari Road, Daryaganj,
New Delhi 110 002, India Phones: +91-11-23272143, +91-11-23272703,
+91-11-23282021, +91-11-23245672, Rel: 32558559
Fax: +91-11-23276490, +91-11-23245683
e-mail: jaypee@jaypeebrothers.com
Visit our website: www.jaypeebrothers.com

Branches

- 2/B, Akruti Society, Jodhpur Gam Road Satellite
Ahmedabad 380 015, Phones: +91-079-26926233, Rel: +91-079-32988717,
Fax: +91-079-26927094 e-mail: jpamdvd@rediffmail.com
- 202 Batavia Chambers, 8 Kumara Krupa Road Kumara Park East,
Bangalore 560 001, Phones: +91-80-22285971, +91-80-22382956,
Rel: +91-80-32714073, Fax: +91-80-22281761 e-mail: jaypeemedpubbgl@eth.net
- 282 IIIrd Floor, Khaleel Shirazi Estate, Fountain Plaza Pantheon Road,
Chennai 600 008, Phones: +91-44-28193265, +91-44-28194897,
Rel: +91-44-32972089, Fax: +91-44-28193231 e-mail: jpchen@eth.net
- 4-2-1067/1-3, 1st Floor, Balaji Building, Ramkote Cross Road
Hyderabad 500 095, Phones: +91-40-66610020, +91-40-24758498,
Rel: +91-40-32940929, Fax: +91-40-24758499, e-mail: jpmedpub@rediffmail.com
- No. 41/3098, B & B1, Kuruvi Building, St. Vincent Road
Kochi 682 018, Kerala, Phones: 0484-4036109
- 1-A Indian Mirror Street, Wellington Square
Kolkata 700 013, Phones: +91-33-22451926, +91-33-22276404, +91-33-22276415,
Rel: +91-33-32901926, Fax: +91-33-22456075, e-mail: jpbcal@dataone.in
- 106 Amit Industrial Estate, 61 Dr SS Rao Road, Near MGM Hospital, Parel,
Mumbai 400 012, Phones: +91-22-24124863, +91-22-24104532,
Rel: +91-22-32926896, Fax: +91-22-24160828,
e-mail: jpmedpub@bom7.vsnl.net.in
- "KAMALPUSHPA" 38, Reshimbag, Opp. Mohota Science College, Umred Road
Nagpur 440 009 (MS) Phones: Rel: 3245220, Fax: 0712-2704275
e-mail: jaypeenagpur@dataone.in

MCQs in Oral and Maxillofacial Pathology

First Edition: **2007**
ISBN 81-8061-859-5
Typeset at JPBMP typesetting unit
Printed at Replika Press Pvt. Ltd.

भारतीय दन्त परिषद

DENTAL COUNCIL OF INDIA

(CONSTITUTED UNDER THE DENTISTS ACT 1948)
Aiwan-E-Galib Marg, Kotla Road, New Delhi-110 002

DR. ANIL KOHLI
MDS (Lko), DNBE (USA)
President DNO-4379
Awardee:
- Padmashri
- Padmabhushan
- Dr.B.C.Roy National Award

Telephone: 23220204 Direct
23238542, 23236740
: 0091 - 11 - 23231252
0091 - 11 - 23220204
E- mail : dciindia@hotmail.com
Website : http://www.dciindia.org

FOREWORD

The progressive concept is changing very fast from subjective to objective. In many universities a part of the professional examination question papers contain objective type questions.

All the competitions contain only Multiple Choice Questions (MCQs). In MCQ type objective question papers, questions from the full course can be covered, while only in subjective type question papers, it is not possible to cover the complete course of the subject, because out of an average of about 50 topics in a subject only 6 questions on 6 topics can be asked. When the question papers are of subjective type, students do only the superficial selective reading and lack the complete and deeper knowledge of the subject. With MCQ type of question papers the chances of leakage of the question papers are also very much reduced as they cover complete course of the subject and the students have to read complete course.

This book provides excellent and comprehensive coverage, covering all the aspects of the subject with unique and to the point explanations, which are in simple and easy language. This book is of great value to the students preparing for BDS and MDS and various competitive examinations.

Dr Anil Kohli
President
Dental Council of India

Preface

This book has been written keeping professional and PG Dental Entrance Examinations in mind. Answers have been given with the explanations. It is based on the experience of many toppers regarding flying success in the examinations. This book will guide in preparations for examination. The questions in this book have been compiled after analyzing many question papers of previous years.

The secret of success in competitive examination lies in proper guidance and hard work. This book simplifies your preparation by making you work more efficiently. For the sake of convenience the MCQs have been divided subjectwise, one book on each major subject. Some allied subjects have been joined together. All the books on MCQs will be true friends and a great asset for the candidates of dental professional examinations, the postgraduate dental entrance examinations and interview and also for practitioners.

The trend is very fast changing toward MCQs. These books will also be very useful for the students of graduate and postgraduate courses, as these contain questions, which are likely to be asked in periodical assessments during graduate and postgraduate courses and in final examinations.

For the preparation for examinations the aim of these books is to encourage the readers to detect areas of weakness in understanding the subject matter so that they may again study the textbooks for better and comprehensive review of the subject.

Every effort has been made to update all the books. All the books will be very useful for all the students and will prepare them to face any examination with full confidence.

Satish Chandra
Shaleen Chandra
Girish Chandra

Tips for Success

1. Start your preparations at least one year in advance. Give six months for initial preparation (Reading textbooks and solving MCQs), 4 months for final preparation (Solving MCQs from books) and last two months for revision of MCQs.
2. Procure all study materials and finish subject by subject.
3. Plan your study hours.
4. Consult your seniors who have passed the examinations with a good score. Follow their advice but not blindly.
5. Read the textbook of the subjects thoroughly from the beginning to the end. Do not do selective reading except only in revision.
6. Be organized in your study.
7. Aim for the top because you will invariably fall short.
8. Practice self-assessment tests and solve model test papers to know which chapters require revision and to get a feel of examination conditions.
9. Understand each chapter of each subject and attempt connected MCQs before proceeding to the next chapter. If you correctly answer less than 90% of MCQs, repeat the chapter.
10. Practise, practise and practise MCQs again and again with reasoning.
11. Time yourself while solving model test papers and examination question papers.
12. Relax and be tension-free while attempting questions in the examination.
13. Read the questions carefully to understand them, think and then answer.

Information and Suggestions

Remember

- You can do it. Always try for the top slots because if you aim for the sky, you would at least reach the hilltop.
- You can do it and have to do it.

Tentative dates of various entrance exams			*Approximate No. of seats available*
All India PG	-	Jan	130
AIIMS	-	Jan/June	4
BHU	-	Jan to March	2
PGI Chandigarh	-	June/Nov	4
MAHE	-	May	50
Various state/ College/ Universities entrances	-	Jan to Dec	1000

The following is the approximate percentage of MCQs appeared in the various postgraduate entrance examinations in previous years.

Subject	*No. of MCQs %age*	*Weeks required for revision*	
		Textbooks	*MCQs books*
1. Purely Preclinical	3	1	1
2. Applied Preclinical	8	2	2
3. Oral and Dental Pathology and Oral Medicine	25	5	5
4. Oral and Maxillofacial Surgery	9	2	2
5. Periodontics	5	1	1
6. Prosthodontics and Applied Dental Material	14	3	3
7. Conservative Dentistry	8	2	2
8. Orthodontics	8	2	2
9. Dental Radiology	3	2	2
10. Endodontics	5	2	2
11. Community Dentistry	2	1	1

Contd...

Contd...

Subject	No. of MCQs %age	Weeks required for revision	
		Textbooks	MCQs books
12. Gen. Medicine and Surgery	5	1	1
13. Pedodontics and Preventive Dentistry	5	1	1
Total	100	25	25

1. Only hard labor and vast knowledge are not enough but mastering the technique of taking MCQs examination is equally important.
2. First, clear the basic fundamentals to have wider and better understanding of the subject. You must read the textbooks as much as possible.
3. Do not attempt the questions that you are not sure of. Negative marks due to guesswork always take you down in the merit list. Even 1 mark can change your merit tremendously.
4. It is better to leave a question rather than to attempt it wrongly.
5. Research in psychology has concluded that most of us mark the right choice first and due to second thoughts mark a wrong choice.
6. The entrance examinations are to test the basic fundamental knowledge of the subject. Mostly the choices are straight forward and not to trick you. Answer each question from general principles rather than from exceptions.
7. Appear in all the entrance examinations in which you are eligible. You never know when luck may favor you.

Contents

1

Developmental Disturbances of Oral and Paraoral Structures

1. Mode of inheritance in hypomaturation of enamel is:

A. Sex linked recessive B. Autosomal dominant
C. Autosomal recessive D. All of the above

2. The origin of most of the developmental anomalies is:

A. Genetic B. Environmental
C. Idiopathic D. None of the above

3. Parry-Romberg syndrome is also known as:

A. Facial hemihypertrophy
B. Micrognathia
C. Macrognathia
D. Facial hemiatrophy

4. All of the following are features of Romberg's syndrome *except*:

A. It generally involves left side of face
B. Electrical stimulus to atrophic facial muscles may be unaltered
C. Jacksonian epilepsy on ipsilateral side occurs
D. It is a form of localized scleroderma

5. van der Woude's syndrome includes:

A. Pits of upper lip and cleft lip and/or cleft palate
B. Pits of upper and lower lip and cleft lip and/or cleft palate
C. Pits of lower lip and cleft lip and/or cleft palate
D. Acquired double lip, blepharochalasis and nontoxic thyroid enlargement

6. **Which of the followings statements about cleft lip and cleft palate is untrue?**
   A. Cleft lip and cleft palate are somewhat more common in boys than in girls
   B. Cleft lip occurs three times more frequently on right side
   C. Boys with cleft lip only have more chance of developing severe defects
   D. Isolated cleft palate is more common in girls

7. **Baelz's disease is:**
   A. Simple type cheilitis glandularis
   B. Superficial suppurative type cheilitis glandularis
   C. Deep suppurative type chelitis glandularis
   D. Myxadenitis labialis

8. **Miescher's syndrome is:**
   A. Cheilitis glandularis
   B. Cheilitis glandularis apostematosa
   C. Baelz's disease
   D. Cheilitis granulomatosa

9. **Which of the following statements is untrue about Peutz-Jeghers syndrome?**
   A. Melanin pigmentation in the form of macules is present from birth
   B. Mucosal pigmentation fades later in life but facial pigmentation persists
   C. Intestinal polyps manifest themselves clinically in the small intestine
   D. It is associated with gastrointestinal carcinoma

10. **Melkersson-Rosenthal syndrome includes:**
   A. Scrotal tongue + Facial paralysis + Cheilitis granulomatosa
   B. Facial paresis + Cheilitis glandularis + Fissured tongue
   C. Acquired double lip+Blepharochalasis + Nontoxic thyroid enlargement
   D. Pits of lower lip and cleft lip and/or cleft palate

11. Beckwith's hypoglycemic syndrome includes all of the followings *except*:

A. Umbilical hernia
B. Postnatal somatic giantism
C. Mild macrocephaly
D. Fetal visceromegaly

12. All of the followings are types of fissured tongue *except*:

A. Transverse
B. Cerebriform
C. Foliaceous
D. Racemose

13. Which of the following papillae are absent in familial dysautonomia?

A. Filiform and circumvallate
B. Filiform and fungiform
C. Fungiform and circumvallate
D. Filiform and foliate

14. Which of the following statements is untrue about hairy tongue?

A. There is hypertrophy of fungiform papillae
B. There is a lack of normal desquamation
C. Sodium peroxide can incite hairy tongue
D. It can be associated with systemic disturbances

15. Which of the following diseases represents Kimura's disease?

A. Lymphoid hamartoma
B. Branchiogenic cyst
C. Eosinophilic lymphoid granuloma
D. Reactive lymphoid hyperplasia

16. Which of the following result in salivary gland enlargement?

A. Menopause B. Starvation
C. Aging process D. All of the above

17. Which of the followings correctly describes atresia?

A. Congenital presence of one or more of the major salivary gland ducts
B. Congenital occlusion of minor salivary gland ducts
C. Widespread distribution of normal accessory salivary glands in the oral cavity
D. Congenital absence of one or more of the major salivary gland ducts

18. What is the location of latent bone cyst?

A. In mid palatine suture
B. Below the mandibular canal
C. Above the mandibular canal
D. Above the mylohyoid ridge

19. Which of the following is always confluent in case of true fusion?

A. Cementum B. Enamel
C. Dentin D. None of the above

20. Fusion of teeth by cementum is known as:

A. Gemination B. Dilaceration
C. Concrescence D. Dens evaginatus

21. Which of the following represent dilacerations?

A. Angulation in the root of a tooth
B. Angulation in the crown of a tooth
C. Sharp bend in the root or crown of a tooth
D. All of the above

22. Talon cusp most commonly involves:

A. Deciduous molars B. Deciduous incisor
C. Permanent incisor D. Permanent premolar

23. Most commonly involved tooth in case of dilated composite odontome is:

A. Deciduous maxillary central incisor
B. Deciduous maxillary lateral incisor
C. Permanent maxillary central incisor
D. Permanent maxillary lateral incisor

24. Leong's premolar is also known as:

A. Dens invaginatus B. Dens evaginatus
C. Occlusal enamel pearl D. Both (B) and (C)

25. Taurodontism shows all of the following features *except*:

A. It occurs in Neanderthal man and also in Klinefelter syndrome patient
B. It more commonly involves permanent teeth
C. It occurs due to failure of Hertwig's epithelial sheath to invaginate at the proper vertical level
D. It most commonly involves molars

26. Anodontia due to multiple unerupted teeth is known as:

A. True anodontia B. False anodontia
C. Pseudoanodontia D. None of the above
Note: (B) is due to extraction of tooth.

27. Most common supernumerary tooth in deciduous dentition is:

A. Maxillary fourth molar B. Mesiodens
C. Maxillary paramolar D. Maxillary lateral incisor

28. Gardner's syndrome shows all of the following features *except*:

A. Epidermoid cyst B. Sebaceous cyst
C. Branchial cyst D. Desmoid tumors

29. Which of the following mechanisms occur in case of hypomaturation type of amelogenesis imperfecta?

A. Disturbance in the differentiation or viability of ameloblast
B. Defects of matrix structure and of mineral deposition
C. Alterations in enamel rod and rod sheath structures
D. None of the above

30. The type/s of enamel hypoplasia due to exanthematous fever is/are:

A. Pitting type B. Change in shape
C. Neonatal ring or line type D. All of the above

31. Which of the following is/are correct statement(s)?

A. Enamel hypoplasia due to hypocalcemia is of pitting type

B. Tooth shows hypoplasia due to local infection or trauma and is known as Turner's tooth

C. Hydrogen peroxide is used for bleaching of mottled enamel

D. All of the above

32. All of the following statements are correct about hereditary opalescent dentin *except*:

A. Type I dentinogenesis imperfecta is associated with osteogenesis Imperfecta

B. Type II dentinogenesis imperfecta shows total precocious obliteration of the pulp chambers and root canals

C. Permanent teeth are more severely affected than deciduous teeth in type I dentinogenesis imperfecta

D. Brandywine type is type III dentinogenesis imperfecta

33. Which of the following statements is correct?

A. Pulp chambers of deciduous teeth in type I dentin dysplasia are wide

B. Periapical radiolucencies occur in type II dentin dysplasia

C. Periapical radiolucencies occur for in type I detin dysplasia involving otherwise intact teeth

D. "Lava flowing around boulders" occurs in case of coronal dentin dysplasia

34. "Thistle-tube" appearance is seen in:

A. Type II (Coronal) dentin dysplasia

B. Type I Radicular dentin dysplasia

C. Regional odontodysplasia

D. Hereditary opalescent dentin

35. All of the followings are correct *except*:

A. Local vascular defects are involved in the pathogenesis of odontogenesis imperfect

B. Most commonly affected tooth in odontogenic dysplasia is permanent maxillary lateral incisor

C. Widening of predentin layer occurs in regional odontodysplasia

D. Rootless teeth are present in dentin dysplasia

36. The teeth erupting prematurely in the first thirty days of life are known as:

A. Deciduous teeth B. Natal teeth

C. Neonatal teeth D. Ghost teeth

37. Most difficult extraction of impacted third molar is of:

A. Horizontal type B. Mesioangular type

C. Distoangular type D. Vertical type

38. Most commonly ankylosed deciduous tooth is:

A. Maxillary 1st molar B. Mandibular 1st molar

C. Mandibular canine D. Mandibular IInd molar

39. Radiographically in which of the following cysts inverted pear shape appearance is present?

A. Median palatal cyst B. Nasoalveolar cyst

C. Globulomaxillary cyst D. Nasopalatine cyst

40. Klestadt's cyst is also known as:

A. Nasopalatine cyst B. Nasoalveolar cyst

C. Both of the above D. Globulomaxillary cyst

41. Which of the following is most common location of thyroglossal tract cyst?

A. Suprahyoid B. Subhyoid

C. Any of above D. Below the cricoid cartilage

42. Which of the following cysts involves bone secondarily?

A. Nasopalatine cyst B. Nasolabial cyst

C. Globulomaxillary cyst D. Epstein's pearl

43. Which of the following types of cleft palate involves only soft palate and may include submucous cleft?

A. Class I B. Class III
C. Class IV D. Class II

Explainations

1.D. Hypomaturation with taurodontism is autosomal dominant, there are also Y-linked recessive and autosomal recessive forms..

2.C. Only about 10 percent of developmental malformations can be explained on genetic basis. The second important factor in the development of such disturbances is that of pathologic environmental conditions, and these have been estimated to account for an additional 10% of developmental anomalies. The remaining 80% are idiopathic.

3.D. Parry-Romberg syndrome is also know as hemifacial atrophy.

4.C. Contralateral Jacksonian epilepsy occurs, other features are as follows. The roots of the teeth may exhibit deficiency of root development and reduced growth of the jaws on the affected side. Eruption of teeth on the affected side may also be retarded.

5.C. Pits may result from notching of lip at an early stage of development, with fixation of tissue at the base of the notch, or from failure of complete union of embryonic lateral sulci of lip, which persist and ultimately develop into typical pits

6.B. Cleft lip occurs about three times more frequently on the left side than on the right.

7.B. Baelz's disease is characterized by painless swelling, induration, crusting, and superficial and deep ulcerations of the lip.

8.D. In cheilitis granulomatosa there is diffuse swelling of the lips, especially the lower lip. This swelling is usually soft and exhibits no pitting upon pressure.

9.B. In Peutz-Jeghers syndrome, facial pigmentation tends to fade later in life, although the mucosal pigmentation persists.

10.A. Although cheilitis granulomatosa may occur without any other manifestation of a disease process, it sometimes appears in association with facial paralysis and scrotal tongue.

11.C. Macroglossia is a prominent feature of Beckwith's hypoglycemic syndrome, which additionally includes neonatal hypoglycemia, mild microcephaly, umbilical hernia, fetal visceromegaly and postnatal somatic giantism.

12.D. Fissured tongue is also known as scrotal tongue.

13.C. The taste buds located in these papillae are also presumable absent, thus explainining the taste deficit in patients with this disease.

14.A. Hairy tongure is characterized by hypertrophy of the filiform papillae.

15.C. Kimura's disease is also known as angio lymphoid hyperplasia with eosinophils, is characterized by are atypical endothelial proliferation with a chronic inflammatory infiltrate, many eosinophils, and aggregates of lymphoid tissue.

16.D. Palatal gland hyperplasia presents as a small localized swelling, measuring from several millimeters to 1 cm, or more in diameter, usually on the hard patate or at the junction of hard and soft palates.

17.D. Atresia may result in the formation of a retention cyst or produce a relatively severe xerostomia.

18.B. Latent bone cyst is generally situated between the mandibular canal and inferior border of the mandible, commonly in the second or third molar area or just anterior to the angle.

19.C. Fusion of teeth is common in the deciduous as well as in the permanent dentition.

20.C. Concrescence occurs as a result of traumatic injury or crowding of teeth with resorption of interdental bone so that the two roots are in approximate contact and become fused by the deposition of cementum between them.

21.D. Dilaceration is thought to be due to trauma during the period in which the tooth is forming, with the result that the position of the calcified portion of the tooth is changed and the remainder of the tooth is formed at an angle.

22.C. The talon cusp, an anomalous structure resembling an eagle's talon, projects lingually from the cingulum areas of a maxillary or mandibular permanent incisor.

23.D. Maxillary central incisors are sometimes involved, and the condition is frequently bilateral.

24.D. The dens evaginatus is a developmental condition that appears clinically as an accessory cusp or globule of enamel on the occlusal surface between the buccal and lingual cusps of premolars, unilaterally or bilaterally.

25.C. In taurodontism, body of the tooth is enlarged at the expense of roots.

26.C. False anodontia is due to extraction of tooth and true anodontia occurs due to congenital absence of teeth.

27.D. The most common supernumerary tooth in permanent dentition, is the mesiodens, a tooth situated between the maxillary central incisors.

28.C. Other features of Gardeners sydrome are multiple polyposis of large intestine, osteomas of long bones, skull and jaws and impacted supernumerary and permanent teeth.

29.C. In hypoplastic type, there is a disturbance in the differentiation or viability of ameloblasts. In the hypocalcification or hypominer alisation type, there are defects of matrix structure and of mineral deposition.

30.A. Teeth involved depend on the timing of fever. If it occurs in first two years then anterior teeth and first molars are affected. However, if it occurs in fourth to fifth year of age then cuspids, bicuspids and second molars are affected. However, teeth most frequently involved are the maxillary central and laterals incisors and maxillary and mandibular premolars.

31.D. Hydrogen peroxide is frequently effective, but the procedure must be carried out periodically, since the teeth continue to stain.

32.C. In general, the deciduous teeth are more severely affected than the permanent teeth in type I.

33.C. Periapical radiolucencies represent either granuloma, cysts or absceses involving vital teeth.

34.A. The permanent teeth exhibit an abnormally large pulp chamber in the coronal portion of the tooth. This is known as thistle tube appearance.

35.B. Maxillary teeth are involved more frequently than the mandibular, the most frequently affected teeth being the maxillary permanent central incisor, lateral incisor and cuspid.

36.C. Teeth present during birth are called natal teeth.

37.C. In distoangular impaction, third molar lies obliquely in the bone, the crown of the tooth pointing distally toward the ramus, the roots approximating the distal root of second molar.

38.D. Submerged teeth are deciduous teeth, most commonly mandibular second molars that have undergone a variable degree of root resorption and then have become ankylosed to the bone.

39.C. This cyst, on intraoral roentgenogram, characteristically appears as an inverted pear shaped radiolucent area between the roots of the maxillary lateral incisor and cuspid, usually causing divergence of the roots of these teeth.

40.B. Nasoalveolar cyst is also known as nasolabial cyst.

41.C. The thyroglossal tract cyst is an uncommon developmental cyst, which may form anywhere along the embryonic thyroglossal tract between the foramen caecum of the tongue and thyroid glands.

42.B. Nasolabial cyst is not found within bone, but is usually described as a rare fissural cyst that nay involves bone secondarily.

43.C. Class I-cleft involving the soft palate and can also be a sub mucous cleft which appears normal it is according Venu (1922).

2

Tumors of Oral Cavity

1. An independent, uncoordinated new growth of tissue which is potentially capable of unlimited growth and does not regress after removal of stimulus is:

A. Tumor
B. Neoplasm
C. Swelling
D. All of the above

2. An exophytic growth of finger like projections and always well circumscribed pedunculated tumor is:

A. Squamous Acanthoma
B. Keratoacanthoma
C. Papilloma
D. None of the above

3. Incidence of breast cancer is increased in:

A. Cowden's syndrome
B. Apert syndrome
C. Treacher-Collins syndrome
D. Crouzon syndrome

4. "Self-healing carcinoma" is:

A. Squamous acanthoma
B. Papilloma
C. Keratoacanthoma
D. Pigmented nevus

5. A lesion which both clinically and histologically resembles epidermoid carcinoma is:

A. Cowden syndrome
B. Keratoacanthoma
C. Squamous acanthoma
D. None of the above

6. Which of the followings is the most common lesion of the skin?

A. Intradermal nevus
B. Junctional nevus
C. Compound nevus
D. Spindle cell nevus

7. Which of the following nevi are extremely common?

A. Congenital nevi
B. Acquired nevi
C. Both of the above
D. None of the above

8. According to most authorities nevus cells are derivatives of:

A. Ectodermal cells
B. Endodermal cells
C. Mesodermal cells
D. Neural crest cells

9. "Dropping-off" or abtropfung effect is shown by:

A. Blue nevus
B. Epithelial cell nevus
C. Junctional nevus
D. Intradermal nevus

10. "Garment nevi" are:

A. Usually 3-5 cm diameter
B. Acquired nevi
C. Greater than 10 cm
D. All of the above

11. Which of the following layers is thickened in acanthosis?

A. Stratum basale
B. Stratum granulosum
C. Stratum corneum
D. Stratum spinosum

12. In which of the following locations, basal cell carcinoma is most frequently found?

A. Middle third of leg
B. Upper third of leg
C. Middle third of face
D. Lower third of face

13. Which of the followings viruses does not cause any human malignant cancer?

A. Herpes simplex virus
B. Varicella zoster virus
C. Epstein Barr virus
D. Cytomegalovirus

14. The parakeratin lining the clefts with the parakeratin plugging is the hallmark of which of the following lesions?

A. Basal cell carcinoma
B. Epidermoid carcinoma
C. Transitional cell carcinoma
D. Verrucous carcinoma

15. Carcinosarcoma is another name of:

A. Verrucous carcinoma
B. Rodent ulcer
C. Spindle cell carcinoma
D. Adenoid squamous cell carcinoma

16. In which of the following cutaneous melanomas only vertical growth phase is present?

A. Lentigo maligna melanoma
B. Superficial spreading melanoma
C. Nodular melanoma
D. Pagetoid melanoma

17. Which of the following combinations is correct regarding metastatic tendency of melanoma?

A. 0.75 cm in thickness and located in body, arm, neck and scalp.
B. 0.75 mm in thickness and located in arm, neck, body and scalp
C. 0.75 cm in thickness and located in back, arm, neck and scalp
C. More than 0.75 mm in thickness and located in arm, neck, back and scalp

18. Most common site of occurrence of giant cell fibroma is:

A. Tongue B. Palate
C. Lip D. Gingiva

19. Most common location of origin of ossifying fibroid epulis is:

A. Tongue B. Buccal mucosa
C. Floor of mouth D. Interdental papilla

20. Which of the following tumors shows variable radiographic finding depending on the stage of development?

A. Giant cell epulis B. Central fibro-osteoma
C. Giant cell fibroma D. Central giant cell granuloma

21. Origin of peripheral giant cell granuloma is:

A. Gingiva B. Interdental papilla
C. Mucoperiosteum D. Tongue

22. Which of the following is a continuation of the normal process of fetal fat development carried into postnatal life?

A. Hibernoma B. Lipoma
C. Lipoblastomatosis D. Fibrolipoma

23. Verruciform xanthoma is also known as:

A. Histiocytosis "Y" B. Histiocytosis "X"
C. Lipoblastomatosis D. Dermatosclerosis

24. Basically, large swollen "foam" cells or xanthoma cells are:

A. Lymphocytes B. Neutrophils
C. Histiocytes D. Eosinophils

25. Most common site of occurrence of hemangioma is:

A. Tongue B. Lip
C. Buccal mucosa D. Floor of mouth

26. "Sun-ray" appearance in radiograph is seen in:

A. Osteosarcoma B. Osteoclastoma
C. Central hemangioma D. None of the above

27. Intramuscular hemangioma arises within:

A. Smooth muscle B. Cardiac muscle
C. Skeletal muscle D. Diseased smooth muscle

28. "Sun-burst" appearance in radiograph is seen in:

A. Osteoclastoma B. Osteosarcoma
C. Central hemangioma D. Both of the above

29. Which of the following consists of an endothelium-lined sac connecting of an artery and a vein?

A. Cirsoid aneurysm B. Varicose aneurysm
C. Aneurysmal varix D. None of the above

30. Which of the followings is wrong about Rendu-Osler-Weber disease?

A. Earliest sign is epistaxis
B. There is lack of elastic fibers in blood vessels
C. There is defect in endothelial cell attachment
D. Both bleeding and clotting time are normal

31. Which of the following nerves is associated with Sturge-Weber disease?

A. Facial nerve
B. Auditory
C. Olfactory
D. Trigeminal

32. Most common site of lymphangioma is:

A. Lips
B. Tongue
C. Palate
D. Buccal mucosa

33. Which of the following is not a division of lymphangioma?

A. Simple lymphangioma
B. Capillary lymphangioma
C. Cavernous lymphangioma
D. Hypertrophic lymphangioma

34. Which of the following types of lymphangioma is most common?

A. Cellular lymphangioma
B. Cystic lymphangioma
C. Diffuse systemic lymphangioma
D. Cavernous lymphangioma

35. Codman's tumor is also known as:

A. Chondroma
B. Myxoma
C. Chondromyxoid fibroma
D. Benign chondroblastoma

36. Gardner's syndrome includes:

A. Chondroma
B. Osteoma
C. Myxoma
D. Chondromyxoid fibroma

37. "Onion-skin" appearance on radiographic film is found in:

A. Endothelial myeloma
B. Osteogenic sarcoma
C. Angioreticuloendothelioma
D. Plasmacytoma

38. Which of the following statements is wrong about "Round cell" sarcoma?

A. Radiographically similar appearance to osteosarcoma if osteophytes are formed.
B. It is extremely cellular neoplasm
C. Presence of multinucleated giant cells
D. Necrosis is a common feature

39. In which of the following diseases symmetrical widening of periodontal ligament space about one or more teeth is found is found on the radiograph?

A. Ewing's sarcoma B. Ehlers-danlos syndrome
C. Osteogenic sarcoma D. Hodgkin's lymphoma

40. "Starry sky" effect seen in African jaw lymphoma is:

A. Radiographic finding B. Clinical finding
C. Histological finding D. None of the above

41. Which of the following is untrue about Burkitt's lymphoma?

A. Its origin is from T-cells
B. It is associated with childhood
C. It primarily involves extranodal tissues
D. Macrophages are responsible for "starry sky" effect

42. Which of the following statements about Hodgkin's disease is wrong?

A. Biomodal age incidence peak is present
B. Lymphocyte depletion type has a localized involvement on one side of the diaphragm
C. Lymphocyte depletion has least favorable prognosis
D. Mixed cellularity has a widespread involvement

43. All of the followings are features of plasmacytoma *except*?

A. Reversal of the serum albumin- globulin ratio occurs
B. Leukemia is a common finding in plasmacytoma
C. Cells show "cartwheel" or "checkerboard" pattern
D. It occurs between the ages of 40-70 years

44. Which of the followings represent a hamartomatous malformation rather than a true neoplasm?

A. Angiomyoma B. Vascular leiomyoma
C. Both of the above D. Leiomyoma

45. Most common site of leiomyosarcoma is:

A. Tongue B. Lip
C. Cheek D. Palate

46. All of the followings are types of rhabdomyosarcoma *except*:

A. Pleomorphic B. Alveolar
C. Capillary D. Embryonal

47. 'Racquet' cells are found in:

A. Leiomyosarcoma
B. Rhabdomyosarcoma
C. Malignant granular cell myoblastoma
D. Liposarcoma

48. All of the following features are present in multiple endocrine neoplasia type I *except*:

A. Tumor of adrenal cortex
B. Peptic ulcers
C. Hyperplasia of parathyroids
D. Medullary carcinoma of thyroid

49. Marfanoid habitus is present in:

A. Multiple endocrine neoplasia type I
B. Multiple endocrine neoplasia type II
C. Multiple endocrine neoplasia type III
D. None of the above

50. Which of the following is most important in relation to prognosis of multiple endocrine neoplasia?

A. Pheochromocytoma of the adrenal medulla
B. Tumors of pituitary gland
C. Peptic ulcer
D. Medullary carcinoma of the thyroid

51. Neurofibroma arises from:

A. Schwann cells B. Fibroblasts
C. Perineurial cells D. All of the above

52. All of the following are malignant transformation of neurofibromatosis *except*:

A. Fibrosarcoma B. Spindle cell sarcoma
C. Neurogenic sarcoma D. Round cell sarcoma

53. Juxtaoral organ of Chievitz is associated with:

A. Greater palatine nerve block
B. Posterior superior alveolar nerve block
C. Inferior alveolar nerve block
D. Infraorbital nerve block

Explanations

1.B. A tumor, by definition, is simply a swelling or enlargement of the tissue; in the strict sense, the word does not imply a neoplastic process. It is one of the cardinal signs of inflammation.

2.C. The papilloma is a common benign neoplasm originating from surface epithelium.

3.A. Cowden's syndrome is an autosomal dominant disease characterized by papillomatous or pebbly lesions in the oral cavity facial trichilemmomas associated with gastrointestinal tract, thyroid, CNS and mucoskeletal abnormalities as well as oral lesions. Breast cancer occurs with relatively high frequency (20 to 36%) in these patients.

4.C. Keretoacanthorma is also known as molluscum pseudocarcinomatosum or verrucoma.

5.B. Keratoacanthoma is a benign epithelial lesion wherewas epidermoid carcinoma is a malignant lesion.

6.A. The common mole may be a smooth flat lesion or may be elevated above the surface, it may or may elevated above the surface, it may or may not exhibit brovon pigmentation, and it often shows strands of hair growing from its surface.

7.B. Acquired nevi appear about the eighth month of life and increase in number with age, apparently reaching their peak numerically in the late third decade of life.

8.D. The nevus cells are large discrete cells, each with an ovoid, vesicular nucleus and pale cytoplasm.

9.C. In Junctional nevus, overlying epithelium is usually thin and irregular and shows cells apparently crossing the junction and growing down into the connective tissue, the so called dropping-off effect.

10.C. The garment nevi are greater than 10 cm in diameter and can cover large areas of the skin.

11.D. Acanthosis may or may not be associated with hyperorthokeratosis or hyperparakeratosis, sometimes occurring independently of changes in the overlying layer.

12.C. This form of carcinoma does not arise from oral mucosa and thus is never seen in the oral cavity unless it arrives there by invasion and infiltration from a skin surface.

13.B. Herpes simplex virus type II causes carcinoma of the uterine cervix. Epstein barr virus causes African jaw (Burkitt's) lymphoma and nasopharyngeal carcinoma. Cytomegalovirus causes Kaposi's sarcoma.

14.D. Even though the lesion may be very extensive, the basement membrane will often appear intact.

15.C. Spindle cell carcinoma is also known as pseudosarcoma or Lane's tumor.

16.C. Vertical growth phase is characterized by the proliferation of malignant epithelioid melanocytas in the underlying connective tissue.

17.D. Melanomas of the upper back, posterolateral arm, neck and posterior scalp tend to have the highest tendency to metastasize and have poor survival rates.

18.D. The most common site of occurrence is gingiva followed by tongue, palate, buccal mucosa and lips.

19.D. It is well demarcated focal mass of tissue on the gingival, with a sessile or pedunculated base. It is of the same color as normal mucosa or slightly reddened.

20.B. In its early stages the central ossifying fibroma paradoxically appears as radiolucent area. As the tumor bone matures, there is increasing calcification and ultimately the lesion has a relatively uniform radiopaque mass.

21.C. It is most often dark red, vascular or hemorrhagic in appearance, and it commonly exhibits surface ulceration.

22.C. It is characterized clinically by the occurence in infants of solitary or multiple soft tissue masses developing at various sites such as the buttock, chest, axilla or neck.

23.A. The lesion has a verrucous, hyperparakeratotic surface showing severe parakeretin plugging. Characteristic feature is presence of foam cells.

24.C. Foam cell fills the connective tissue papillae between the epithelial pegs.

25.B. The most common site of occurrence are the lips, tongue, buccal mucosa and palate. The tumor often is traumatized and undergoes ulceration and secondary infection.

26.A.

27.C. Intramuscular hemangioma arises within normal skeletal muscles, comprises less than 1 percent of all hemangiomas and is important chiefly because of the problem in differential diagnosis and of treatrment of the lesion.

28.B. Some central hemangiomas present a honey combed appearance on the roentgenogram, sometimes with radiating spicules at the expanded periphery mimiking a sun burst appearance. But it is typical of osteosarcoma.

29.B. A cirsoid aneurysm is a tortuous mass of small arteries and veins linking a larger artery and vein. An aneurysmal varix is a direct connection between an artery and a dilated vein.

30.B. Primary intrinsic defect of the endothelial cells permitting their detachment, or a defect in the perivascular supportive tissue bed, which weakens the vessels, rather than a lack of elastic fibres as was thought at one time.

31.D. Sturge-weber disease is also known as encephalotrigeminal angiomatosis.

32.B. The intraoral lymphangioma most commonly occurs on the tongue, but is seen also on the palate, buccal mucosa, gingiva and lips.

33.B. The following divisions are proposed:(i) Simple lymphangioma (ii) Cavernous lymphangioma (iii) Cellular or hypertrophic lymphangioma, (iv) Diffuse systemic lymphangioma, and (v) Cystic lymphangioma or hygroma.

34.D. The lymphangioma, of which the cavernous type is most common, consists of numerous dilated lymphatics, lined by endothelial cells and containing lymph.

35.D. Codman's tumor is also known as epiphyseal chondromatous giant cell tumor or benign chondro-blastoma.

36.B. Multiple osteomas of the jaws, as well as of long bones and skull, are a charcteristic manifestation of gardner's syndrome.

37.A. Endothelial myeloma is also known as Ewing's sarcoma or "Round cell" sarcoma.

38.C. Ewing's sarcoma is an extremely cellular neoplasm composed of solid sheets or masses of round cells with very little stroma, although a few connective tissue septa may be present.

39.C. This feature is also seen in scleroderma or acrosclerosis.

40.C. Macrophages with an abundant clear cytoplasm, often containing cellular debris, are usually found scattered uniformly throughout the tumor, producing the very characteristic "Starry Sky" effect.

41.A. The endemic african form of the disease is confined almost exclusively to children between 2 to 14 years and involves extranodal tissue.

42.B. The lymphocyte predominant type has the most favorable prognosis, followed by nodular sclerosis, mixed cellularity and lymphocyte depletion, the least favorable.

43.B. Many patients, but not all, exhibit a hyperglobulinemia resulting in a reversal of the serum albumin-globulin ratio and an increase in total serum protein to a level of 8 to 16 gm%.

44.C. Solid leiomyoma represents a true neoplasm.

45.C. The leiomyosarcoma is a malignant tumor of smooth muscle orgin.

46.C. The four forms of rhabdomyosarcoma are:(i) Pleomorphic (ii) Alveolar (iii) Embryonal and (iv) Botryoid.

47.B. A characteristic feature of this form of tumor is the large bizarre cells, the nuclei situated often in an expanded end of the cells, the "recquet cell".

48.D. Medullary carcinoma of thyroid is a feature of MEN type II.

49.C. MEN III is characterized by mucocutaneous neuromas, pheochroma cytomas of the adrenal medulla, medullary carcinoma of thyroid and frequently a marfanoid habitus.

50.D. The most important aspect of this syndrome is the medullary carcinoma of the thyroid because of its ability to metastasize and cause death.

51.D. The neurofibroma is a tumor of nerve tissue origin.

52.D. The great clinical significance of neurofibromatosis lies in the fact that in some patients malignant transformation subsequently occurs in one or more of their lesion.

53.C. Juxtaoral organ of chievitz is a cluster of nests of squamous epithelial cells, sometimes with a duct like appearance, found microscopically in tissue taken from approximate site used by the dentist for injection of inferior alveolar nerve.

3

Tumors of Salivary Glands

1. Among the following, which is the most common site of occurrence of intraoral accessory salivary gland tumors?

A. Hard palate B. Soft palate
C. Cheek D. Tongue

2. Which of the following is also known as 'mixed' tumor?

A. Warthin's tumor
B. Oncocytoma
C. Carcinoma explemorphic adenoma
D. Pleomorphic adenoma

3. Among the following, which is the most common site of occurrence of pleomorphic adenoma?

A. Hard palate B. Soft palate
C. Parotid gland D. Submaxillary gland

4. Which of the following tumors originates from intercalated duct or reserve cell?

A. Pleomorphic adenoma
B. Monomorphic adenoma
C. Canalicular adenoma
D. Basal cell adenoma

5. Which of the following tumors originates primarily from intraoral accessory salivary gland and mostly occurs in upper lip?

A. Basal cell adenoma B. Canalicular adenoma
C. Oncocytoma D. Warthin's tumor

6. "Party wall" appearance is found in:

A. Warthin's tumor B. Canalicular adeonoma
C. Basal cell adenoma D. Pleomorphic adenoma

7. **Which of the following tumors occurs almost exclusively in parotid gland?**
   A. Acidophilic adenoma
   B. Myoepithelioma
   C. Pleomorphic adenoma
   D. Adenolymphoma

8. **The cell present in connective tissue papillae of Sialadenoma papilliferum is:**
   A. Lymphocyte B. Plasma cell
   C. Giant cell D. Basophil

9. **The origin of benign lymphoepithelial lesion is:**
   A. Hereditary B. Environmental
   C. Autoimmune D. None of the above

10. **Which of the following could not be present in Sjögren's syndrome?**
   A. Systemic lupus erythematosus
   B. Polyarteritis nodosa
   C. Polymyositis
   D. None of the above

11. **Radiographically "branchless fruit-laden tree" is present in:**
   A. Mikulicz's disease B. Sjögren's disease
   C. Cylindroma D. Acinic cell carcinoma

12. **In which of the following carcinomas palatal mucosa is a common site of occurrence?**
   A. Acinic cell carcinoma
   B. Basaloid mixed tumor
   C. Mucoepidermoid carcinoma
   D. Sjögren's syndrome

13. **Spread of tumor cells along perineural sheath occurs in:**
   A. Cylindroma
   B. Acinic cell carcinoma
   C. Mucoepidermoid carcinoma
   D. Mucoepithelioma

14. Which of the following tumors arises from cells of terminal salivary gland ducts?

A. Clear cell carcinoma
B. Necrotizing sialometaplasia
C. Acinic cell carcinoma
D. Mucoepidermoid carcinoma

15. Which of the following is not a growth pattern for acinic cell carcinoma?

A. Solid B. Microcytic
C. Follicular D. Cavernous

16. Which of the followings is most common malignant salivary gland tumor of children?

A. Epidermoid carcinoma
B. Acinic cell carcinoma
C. Clear cell carcinoma
D. Mucoepidermoid carcinoma

17. Which of the following statements is untrue about necrotizing sialometaplasia?

A. Most common site is palate
B. It is generally present as an ulcer
C. It is a benign, noninflammatory reaction of salivary gland tissue
D. It commonly develops after the administration of greater palatine nerve block

18. Which of the following statements is untrue about clear cell carcinoma?

A. All clear cell tumors are of high grade malignancy
B. Donath-seifert tumor is a type of clear cell carcinoma
C. Clusters of clear cells present in a pentagonal arrangement
D. None of the above

19. Which of the following patterns do(es) not influence the prognosis of adenoid cystic carcinoma?

A. Site of occurrence B. Histological pattern
C. Both of the above D. None of the above

20. In most cases Sjögren's syndrome is treated by:

A. Surgical excision
B. Radiotherapy
C. Both of the above
D. Symptomatic treatment

Explanations

1.A. Salivary gland tumor are much more common on the hard palete than on the soft, probably there are a greater number of gland aggregates on the hard palate than on the soft palate.

2.D. The term "pleomorphic adenoma"suggested by Willis characterizes closely the unusal histologic pattern of the lesion.

3.C. The most common site of occurence of pleomorphic adenoma is parotid gland.

4.D. Intercalated duct or reserve cell is the histogenetic source of basal cell adenoma.

5.B. The canalicular adenoma is a distinctive variant of the monomorphic adenoma.

6.B. The canalicular adenoma has a strikingly characteristic picture. It is composed of long strands or cords of epithelial cels, almost invariable arranged in a double row and usually showing a "party wall."

7.D. Adenolymphoma is generally superficial, lying just bencath the parotid capsule or protruding through it. It is not painful, is firm to palpation and is clinically indistinguishable from other benign lesions of the parotid gland.

8.B. The lesion is treated by simple surgical excision.

9.C. Benign lymphoepithelial lesion is also known as Mikulicz's disease.

10.D. Sjögren's syndrome is a condition originally described as a triad consisting of keratouconjunctivitis sicca, xerostomia and rheumatoid arthritis.

11.B. Sialographs demonstrate the formation of punctate, cavitary defects, which are filled with radiopaque contrast media. These filling defects have been said to produce "Cherry blossom"or "branchless fruit-laden tree."

12.B. Basaloid mixed tumor is also known as adenoid cystic carcinoma.

13.A. It is of interest that despite the malignant nature of the lesion, mitotic figures are extremely rare.

14.C. The acinic cell carcinoma closely resembles the pleomorphic adenoma in gross appearance, tending to be encapsulated and lobulated.

15.D. Growth patterns for acinic cell carcinoma includes (i) Solid, (ii) Papillary-cystic (iii) Follicular and (iv) Microcystic.

16.D. Mucoepidermoid carcinoma occurs with an equal distribution between men and women .It occurs primarily in the third to fifth decades of life.

17.C. Necrotizing sialometaplasia is a benign, inflammatory reaction of salivary gland tissue which both clinically and histologically mimics a salivary gland malignancy.

18.A. Clear cell carcinomas are composed of clusters of cells surrounded by thin septa of fibrous connective tissue. This often produces somewhat of an "organoid"appearance.

19.D. Site of occurrence is parotid glamd or submaxillary gland or accessory glands on palate and tongue. The stromal connective tissue becomes hyalinized and surrounds the tumor cells, forming a structural pattern of cylinders from which the lesion originally derived the name "cylindroma."

20.D. Keratoconjunctivitis is treated by instillation of ocular lubricants such as artificial tears containing methylcellulose, and xerostomia is treated by saliva substitutes such as those used in treatment of persons with xerostomia secondary to radiation therapy.

4

Cysts and Tumors of Odontogenic Origin

1. Which of the following cysts is formed in place of tooth?

A. Dentigerous cyst
B. Eruption cyst
C. Odontogenic keratocyst
D. Primordial cyst

2. Highest recurrence rate is found in:

A. Primordial cyst B. Odontogenic keratocyst
C. Dentigerous cyst D. Periapical cyst

3. Rushton bodies within the lining epithelium is present in:

A. Periapical cyst
B. Primordial cyst
C. Dentigerous cyst exhibiting inflammation
D. Gingival cyst

4. From which of the following ameloblastoma arises in case of dentigerous cyst?

A. From lining epithelium
B. From rests of odontogenic epithelium in the wall of the cyst
C. Both of the above
D. From rest cells of malassez

5. Which of the followings can arise from dentigerous cyst?

A. Ameloblastoma
B. Epidermoid carcinoma
C. Mucoepidermoid carcinoma
D. All of the above

6. Botryoid odontogenic cyst is a type of:

A. Gingival cyst of new born
B. Gingival cyst of adult
C. Apical periodontal cyst
D. Lateral periodontal cyst

7. Epstein's pearls are found:

A. At the junction of hard and soft palate
B. Along the midpalatine raphe
C. At the region of incisive papillae
D. On the soft palate

8. All of the following are characteristic of odontogenic keratocyst *except*:

A. Parakeratinized surface which is typically corrugated
B. Basal layer of cells shows a "picket fence" or "tombstone" appearance
C. Thickness of epithelium ranges from six to ten cells thick
D. None of the above

9. Which of the following is untrue about odontogenic keratocyst?

A. Most important feature is its high recurrence rate
B. It can develop into epidermoid carcinoma
C. High recurrence is due to inaccurate method of treatment
D. In maxilla, second most common site after third molar area is cuspid area

10. Gorlin and Goltz syndrome is also known as:

A. Hereditary cutaneomandibular polyoncosis
B. Basal cell nevus syndrome
C. Both of the above
D. None of the above

11. All of the following abnormalities are included in Gorlin and Goltz syndrome *except*:

A. Sexual abnormality
B. Dental anomalies
C. Organ abnormality
D. Ophthalmologic abnormality

12. "Ghost" cells are present in:

A. Dentigerous cyst
B. Periapical cyst
C. Primordial cyst
D. Calcifying odontogenic cyst

13. All of the following can give rise to ameloblastoma *except*:

A. Odontoma
B. Basal cells of the surface epithelium of the jaws
C. Remnants of Hertwig's sheath
D. None of the these

14. Most of the peripheral ameloblastoma is:

A. Cystic type
B. Follicular type
C. Acanthomatous type
D. Simple type

15. Pituitary ameloblastoma is also known as:

A. Craniopharyngioma
B. Rathke's pouch tumor
C. Both of the above
D. Medullary carcinoma

16. Least common type of ameloblastoma is:

A. Follicular ameloblastoma
B. Plexiform ameloblastoma
C. Acanthomatous ameloblastoma
D. Basal cell ameloblastoma

17. Pindborg tumor and ameloblastoma are similar in:

A. Patient's age group
B. Radiographic appearance
C. Both of the above
D. Histologic features

18. Radiographically "driven snow" appearance is found in:

A. Adenomatoid odontogenic tumor
B. Benign epithelial odontogenic tumor
C. Calcifying epithelial odontogenic tumor
D. Peripheral odontogenic fibroma

19. Liesegang rings type of calcification is found in:

A. Adenoameloblastoma
B. Calcifying fibrous epulis
C. Central odontogenic fibroma
D. Calcifying epithelial odontogenic tumor

20. Which of the following is the source of epithelial cells in Pindborg tumor?

A. Reduced enamel epithelium
B. Stratum intermedium
C. Stellate reticulum
D. Stratum basale

21. Which of the following is untrue about adenoameloblastoma?

A. It generally involves younger age group patients
B. It more commonly involves mandible in relation to maxilla
C. Most commonly unerupted tooth associated with this is maxillary cuspid
D. Radiographically, in majority of cases it resembles a dentigerous cyst

22. Most common site of occurrence of adenomatoid odontogenic tumor is:

A. Maxillary ramus area
B. Maxillary cuspid area
C. Mandibular premolar area
D. Maxillary anterior area

23. Squamous odontogenic tumor histologically resembles:

A. Follicular ameloblastoma
B. Plexiform ameloblastoma
C. Unicystic ameloblastoma
D. Acanthomatous ameloblastoma

24. Odontogenic tumor having most poorly defined parameters is:

A. Odontogenic myxoma
B. Squamous odontogenic tumor
C. Peripheral odontogenic fibroma
D. Central odontogenic fibroma

25. Which of the following chemicals is associated with neoplastic behaviour of odontogenic myxoma?

A. Chondroitin sulfate
B. Glucose-6-phosphate
C. Hyaluronic acid
D. Acetic acid

26. Most commonly involved tooth in periapical cemental dysplasia is:

A. Mandibular first molar
B. Mandibular third molar
C. Maxillary cuspid
D. Mandibular incisor

27. Varying radiographic appearance is found in:

A. True cementoma
B. Central cementifying fibroma
C. Cementoblastoma
D. Gigantiform cementoma

28. Which of the following stages of periapical cemental dysplasia is radiographically similar to condensing osteitis?

A. Mature stage
B. Cementoblastic stage
C. Osteolytic stage
D. Earliest stage of development

29. Which of the following lesions shows linear growth pattern?

A. Central cementifying fibroma
B. Central cemento-ossifying fibroma
C. Fibrous dysplasia
D. Central ossifying fibroma

30. All of the following are true about benign cementoblastoma *except*:

A. It is a true neoplasm of functional cementoblasts
B. Maxilla is affected more commonly
C. Mostly permanent mandibular first molar is involved
D. Associated tooth is vital

31. All of the following are true about ameloblastic fibroma *except*:

A. It occurs most commonly in mandibular molar area
B. It exhibits fast clinical growth and tends to infiltrate
C. The cells resemble more to dental lamina than to ameloblastoma
D. It occurs in younger age group patient

32. Most common complaint of ameloblastic fibro-odontoma is:

A. Failure of tooth eruption
B. Pain
C. Pus discharge
D. None of the above

33. Calcified tissue bearing no morphological similarity to tooth is known as:

A. Compound composite odontoma
B. Complex composite odontoma
C. Odontoma
D. Composite odontoma

34. Which of the following statements is correct?

A. Compound odontoma is less common than complex odontoma
B. Both types of odontoma have a predilection for right side of the jaw
C. Ghost cells are absent in odontomas
D. Majority of odontoma in the anterior segment of the jaws are complex composite odontomas

35. Complex composite odontomas are common in:

A. Anterior portion of maxilla
B. Posterior portion of maxilla
C. Anterior portion of mandible
D. None of the above

36. Which of the following tumors is frequently malignant?

A. Ameloblastic odontoma
B. Composite odontoma
C. Complex odontoma
D. Testicular teratoma

37. Most common age of occurrence of ameloblastic fibro-odontoma is:

A. 10-15 years age group B. 30-40 years age group
C. 50-55 years age group D. Above 75 year

38. Which of the following cysts involves bone secondarily?

A. Nasopalatine cyst B. Nasolabial cyst
C. Globulomaxillary cyst D. Epstein's pearl

Explanations

1.D. Primordial cyst develops through cystic degeneration and liquefaction of the stellate reticulum in an enamel organ before any calcified enamel or dentin has been formed. Thus the primordial cyst is found in place of a tooth.

2.B. Rcerurence occurs due to thin and friable living of the cyst, which easily breaks during removal.

3.C. These are peculiar linear, often cured, hyaline bodies with variable stainability which are of uncertain origin, questionable nature and unknown significance.

4.C. Development of epidermoid carcinoma also occurs from lining epithelium or from rests of odontogenic epithelium in the wall of the cyst.

5.D. The development of a mucoepidermoid carcinoma occurs from the lining epithelium of the dentigerous cyst which contains mucus secreting cells. Also refer to answer No. 4.

6.D. Botryoid odontogenic cyst is simply a polycystic variant of the lateral periodontal cyst developing through cystic transformation of multiple islands of dental lamina rests.

7.B. Epstein's pearls are cystic, keratin filled nodules found along the mid palatine raphe, probably derived from entrapped epithelial remnants along the line of fusion.

8.D. Common features are pain, soft tissue swelling and expansion of bone, drainage and various neurologic manifestations such as paresthesia of the lip or teeth.

9.C. Recurrence of the keratocyst is due to the nature of the lesion itself, i.e. the presence of additional remnants of dental lamina from which a cyst may develop, and is not related to its method of treatment.

10.C. Gorlin and Goltz syndrome is also known as jaw cyst basal cell nevus-bifid rib syndrome.

11.C. Cutaneous anomalies and neurologic anomalies are also present in Gorlin and Goltz syndrome.

12.D. Ghost cells are pale, eosinophilic, swollen epithelial cells that have lost the nucleus but show a faint outline of the cellular and nuclear membrane.

13.D. Epithelium of odontogenic cysts and disturbances of the developing enamel organ can also give rise to ameloblastoma.

14.C. Peripheral ameloblastoma histologically resembles the typical central or intraosseous ameloblastoma but which occurs in the soft tissue outside and overlying the alveolar bone.

15.C. This is a neoplasm involving the central nervous system which grows as a pseudoencapsulated mass usually in the suprasellar area but occasionally in the intrasellar area, and often destroys the pituatary gland.

16.D. The basal cell type of ameloblastoma bears wnsiderable resemblance to the basal cell carinoma of the skin.

17.A. The averge age of the patient at the time of discovery of the ameloblastic lesion is approximately 33 years, while the average duration of the tumor after discovery is approximately six years Pindborg tumor also occurs in middle aged individuals.

18.C. Scattered flecks of calcification throughout the radiolucency have given rise to the descriptive term of a "driven snow" apearence.

19.D. Calcification actually appears to occur in some instances in globules of the anyloid-like material many of which have coalesced and are transformed from being PAS negative to PAS positive.

20.B. Tumor cell are morphologically similar to the normal cells of stratum intermedium of the odontogenic apparatus.

21.B. The site of occurrence is greater in the maxilla (65 percent) than in the mandible (35 percent).

22.D. In contrast to the ameloblastoma, this tumor occurs mone frequently in the anterior part of the jaws with 76 percent developing anterior to the cuspid in the maxilla and mandible.

23.D. The squamous odontogenic tumor is composed entirely of islands of mature squamous epithelium without a peripheral palisaded or polarized columnar layer.

24.D. Central odontogenic fibroma is a fibroblastic neoplasm containing varying amounts of odontogenic epithelium and, in some cases, calcified material resembling dysplastic dentin or cementum-like material.

25.C. Two acid mucopolysaccharides are reported in the odontogenic myxoma: relatively large quantities of hyaluronic acid and lesser amounts of chondroitin sulfate.

26.D. The lesion occurs in and near the periodontal ligament around the apex of a tooth, usually a mandibular incisor.

27.B. The neoplasm presents an extremely variable roentgenographic appearance depending upon its stage of development.

28.A. In mature stage, an excessive amount of calcified material is deposited in the focal area and appears on the roentgenogram as a well defined radiopacity that is usually bordered by thin radiolucent line or band.

29.C. The central cementifying fibroma and its related lesions, the central ossifying fibroma and central cemento-occifying fibroma, have a centrifugal growth pattern rather than a linear one.

30.B. Mandible is afftected three times more frequently than the maxilla.

31.B. Ameloblastic fibroma exhibits somewhat slower clinical growth than simple ameloblastoma and does not tend to infiltrate between trabeculae of bone.

32.A. Clinical manifestations of the lesion are often absent. The two most common presenting complaints are swelling and failure of tooth eruption.

33.B. In compound composite odontomas, there is at least superficial anatomic similarity to normal teeth.

34.B. Odontoma is a growth in which both the epithelial cells and mesenchymal cells exhibit complete differentiation, with the result that functional ameloblasts and odontoblasts form enamel and dentin.

35.B. In general, complex odontomas had a predilection for the posterior jaws (59%) and lastly the premolar area (7%).

36.D. The teratoma is a ture neoplasm made up of a number of different types of tissue which are not native to the area in which the tumor occurs.

37.A.

38.B. The nasolabial cyst; also called as nasoalveolar cyst is not found within bone, but is usually descrided as a rare fissural cyst that may involve bone secondarily.

5

Regressive Changes of Teeth

1. In normal occlusion, wear facet on the lingual surface of a maxillary canine can be caused by:

A. Mandibular canine only
B. Mandibular first premolar only
C. Mandibular canine and first premolar
D. Mandibular canine and lateral incisor

2. With age, the alteration in size of pulp chamber is a direct result of:

A. Deposition of primary dentin
B. Deposition of secondary dentin
C. Pulp fibrosis
D. Metaplasia

3. Attrition is:

A. Physiologic wearing of a tooth
B. Pathologic wearing away of a tooth surface through some abnormal mechanical process
C. Loss of tooth substance by a chemical process
D. May be physiologic or pathologic

4. Incisal wear of anterior teeth increases the ratio of lingual surface crown length to labial surface crown length in:

A. Maxillary canines only
B. Mandibular canines only
C. All maxillary anterior teeth
D. All mandibular anterior teeth

5. In patients with anorexia nervosa, the condition commonly seen is:

A. Attrition
B. Abrasion
C. Erosion
D. Dentinal Sclerosis

6. Generalized hypercementosis is characteristically seen in:

A. Fibrous dysplasia
B. Paget's disease
C. Hyperparathyroidism
D. Cherubism

7. Primary dentin has:

A. Fewer tubules than secondary dentin
B. More number of tubules than secondary dentin
C. Same number of tubules as secondary dentin
D. None of the above

8. Dead tracts appear:

A. Black in transmitted light
B. Black in reflected light
C. White in transmitted light
D. Same in both transmitted and reflected lights

9. Sclerotic dentin appears:

A. Transparent in reflected light
B. Dark in reflected light
C. Dark in transmitted light
D. None of the above

10. The most common cause of abrasion is:

A. Use of abrasive dentifrices
B. Habit of holding pins between teeth
C. Pipe smoking
D. Use of dental floss

11. Abrasion is most commonly seen on:

A. Occlusal surface
B. Proximal surface
C. Exposed root surface
D. Equally on all surfaces

12. Erosion is most frequently found on:

A. Lingual surfaces
B. Facial surfaces
C. Proximal surfaces
D. Incisal or occlusal surfaces

13. People who frequently consume carbonated beverages or lemon juice are affected by:

A. Dentinal sclerosis
B. Attrition
C. Abrasion
D. Erosion

14. The notches of the incisal edge of the maxillary central incisor due to habitual holding of pin in the mouth is an example of:

A. Attrition
B. Abrasion
C. Erosion
D. None of the above

15. If the cemental overgrowth improves the functional qualities of the cementum it is called:

A. Cementum hypertrophy
B. Cementum hyperplasia
C. Cementum metaplasia
D. Cementum hypoplasia

16. The cementum that is first to be formed is:

A. Cellular cementum
B. Acellular cementum
C. Both are simultaneously formed
D. None of the above

17. Regressive changes in pulp are:

A. Decrease in number of cellular elements
B. Increase in number of collagen fibers
C. Pulpal calcifications
D. All of the above

18. Factor/s that may cause the need for restoration of teeth is/are:

A. Caries
B. Abrasion
C. Attrition
D. All of the above

19. Attrition is characterized by:

A. Occlusal wear only
B. Proximal wear only
C. Both occlusal and proximal wear
D. None of the above

20. Which of the following diseases is associated with erosion?

A. Anorexia nervosa
B. Bulimia
C. Gastro-oesophageal reflux
D. All of the above

21. A condition that develops as a result of horizontal brushing is:

A. Attrition B. Abrasion
C. Erosion D. No effect

22. During tooth resorption there is:

A. Continuous resorption only
B. Resorption only in an episodic phase
C. Resorption and deposition alternately
D. Any of the above

23. 'Pink tooth' is associated with which of the following?

A. Traumatic occlusion B. Internal resorption
C. Pulpal hyperemia D. Periapical granuloma

24. When force is exerted on tooth:

A. Bone resorbs faster than cementum
B. Cementum resorbs faster than bone
C. Both resorb at the same rate
D. Only resorption of bone occurs

25. Which of the following is/are true about tertiary dentin?

A. It is called reparative dentin
B. It is localized exclusively adjacent to irritated zone
C. Tubules are irregular and tortuous
D. All of the above

26. If the cemental overgrowth occurs in non-functional teeth, it is termed as:

A. Hypertrophy B. Hyperplasia
C. Metaplasia D. Aplasia

27. Transverse fracture of root heals by:

A. Formation of new cementum
B. Formation of dentin
C. Bone formation at the site of fracture
D. Formation of dentin and bone

28. Treatment of hypercementosis involves:

A. Extraction of tooth
B. Root canal therapy
C. Removal of calcified masses
D. No treatment required

Explanations

1.C. The first clinical manifestation of attrition may be the appearance of small polished facet on a cusp tip or ridge or a slight flattening of an incisal edge.

2.B. The rate of secondary dentin deposition is usually sufficient to preclude the possibility of pulp exposure through attrition alone.

3.A. Attrition may be defined as the physiologic wearing away of a tooth as a result of tooth- to-tooth contact, as in mastication.

4.D. There is also shortening of the length of the dental arch due to reduction in the mesiodistal diameters of the teeth through proximal attrition.

5.C. Anorexia nervosa is a psychosomatic disease, which is characterized by induced chronic vomiting, often after bouts of uncontrolled eating that are interspersed between periods of starvation because of an inner rejection of food.

6.B. Paget's disease of bone is a generalized skeletal disease characterized by deposition of excessive amounts of secondary cementum on the roots of the teeth and by the apparent disappearance of the lamina dura of teeth.

7.B. Secondary dentin arising in response to irritation is usually irregular in nature, being composed of few tubules which may be tortuous in appearance.

8.A. This optical phenomenon is due to difference in the refractive indices of the affected tubules and normal tubules.

9.B. Dyes do not penetrate those dentinal tubules that are sclerotic as a result either of age or of a slowly progressive type of dental caries.

10.A. Although modern dentifrices are not sufficiently abrasive to damage intact enamel severely, they can cause remarkable wear of cementum and dentin if the tooth brush carring the dentifrice is injudiciously used.

11.C. Abrasion usually occurs on the exposed root surfaces of teeth, but under certain circumstances it may be seen else where, such as on incisal or proximal surfaces.

12.B. Erosion is defined as a loss of tooth substance by a chemical process that does not involve known bacterial action.

13.D. Surface most commonly affected by carbonated beverages or lemon juice are labial surfaces.

14.B. Habitual pipe smokers may develop notching of the teeth that conforms to the shape of the pipe stem.

15.A. Hyperplasia may be regarded as a regressive change of teeth characterized by the deposition of excessive amounts of secondary cementum on root surfaces.

16.B.

17.D. Regressive changes in pulp also include presence of large vacuolated spaces in the pulp.

18.D.

19.C. Attrition occurs only on the occlusal, incisal and proximal surfaces of teeth, not on other surfaces unless a very unusual occlusal relation or malocclusion exists.

20.D. In cases of chronic vomiting, the lingual surfaces of the teeth, particularly of the anterior teeth may exhibit complete loss of enamel through dissolution by gastric hydrochloric acid.

21.B. Abrasion is more common on the left side of the mouth in right- handed people, and vice versa, suggest that improper tooth brushing cause abrasion.

22.C.

23.B. The first evidence of internal resorption is the appearance of pink hued area on the crown of the tooth, which represents the hyperplastic, vascular pulp tissue filling the resorbed area and showing through the remaining overlying tooth substance.

24.D. Bone undergoes resorption for more readily than cementum when force is exerted upon the tooth by orthodontic appliances or by occlusal trauma.

25.D. Irregular dentin, reparative dentin and irritation dentin are synonyms of tertiary dentin.

26.B. Thickness of cementum is increased in non- functional teeth, including embedded or impacted teeth.

27.A. Root fracture is also repaired on occasion by deposition of cementum between the root fragments as well as on their periphery.

28.D. The extraction of teeth because of hypercementosis is contraindicated, since the prognosis of such teeth is excellent in absence of concomitant infection.

6

Bacterial, Viral and Mycotic Infections

1. Scarlet fever is caused by:

A. Staphylococcal organism of the beta-hemolytic type
B. Staphylococcal organism of the alpha-hemolytic type
C. Streptococcal organism of the beta-hemolytic type
D. Streptococcal organism of the alpha-hemolytic type

2. Incubation period of scarlet fever is:

A. Five to ten days
B. One to two weeks
C. Twelve to twenty-one days
D. Three to five days

3. "Strawberry tongue" is a feature of:

A. Diphtheria
B. Tuberculosis
C. Scarlet fever
D. Heerfordt's syndrome

4. Which of the following is not a characteristic of scarlet fever?

A. Skin rashes are prominent in skin folds
B. Raspberry tongue appears before strawberry tongue
C. In strawberry tongue, fungiform papillae appear as small red knobs
D. Meningitis is a complication of scarlet fever

5. Klebs-Löffler bacillus is a:

A. Gram-negative bacillus
B. Gram-negative coccus
C. Gram-positive bacillus
D. Gram-positive coccus

6. Which of the following areas is used as entry area of microorganism in case of scarlet fever?

A. Upper respiratory tract B. Lower respiratory tract
C. Pharynx D. Oral cavity

7. Most common site of involvement of oral mucous membrane in case of tuberculosis is:

A. Tongue B. Palate
C. Lips D. Gingiva

8. Scrofula is tuberculous infection of:

A. Parotid lymph nodes
B. Submaxillary and cervical lymph nodes
C. Submandibular and cervical lymph nodes
D. Apex of lungs

9. Etiology of sarcoidosis is:

A. Corynebacterium diphtheriae
B. Mycobacterium bovis
C. Pasteurella tularensis
D. None of the above

10. Kveim-siltzbach test is used for:

A. Uveoparotid fever B. Sarcoidosis
C. Tuberculosis D. Leprosy

11. Most common nerve involvement in case of Heerfordt's syndrome is:

A. Unilateral trigeminal nerve paralysis
B. Bilateral trigeminal nerve paralysis
C. Unilateral or bilateral facial nerve paralysis
D. Unilateral olfactory nerve paralysis

12. Hansen's disease is also known as:

A. Tuberculosis B. Leprosy
C. Sarcoidosis D. Uveoparotid fever

13. Which of the following bacteria produces "Lumpy jaw"?

A. *Actinomyces israelii* B. *Actinomyces naeslundi*
C. *Actinomyces viscous* D. *Actinomyces bovis*

14. "Sulfur granules" are characteristic feature of:

A. Leprosy
B. Actinomycosis
C. Sarcoidosis
D. Syphilis

15. All of the followings are true about actinomycosis *except*:

A. It is an opportunistic infection
B. Most common type of actinomycosis is cervicofacial type
C. Trauma seems to play a role in some cases of actinomycosis
D. It is not a communicable disease

16. Rabbit fever is caused by:

A. *Pseudomonas pseudomallei*
B. *Pasteurella tularensis*
C. *Calymmatobacterium granulomatis*
D. *Klebsiella rhinoscleromatis*

17. General sequence of events in case of tularemia is known as:

A. Oculoglandular tularemia
B. Ulceroglandular tularemia
C. Tularemic pneumonia
D. Pleuritis

18. "Lock-jaw" is caused by:

A. Endotoxin of the *Clostridium tetani*
B. Tetanospasmin of the *Clostridium tetani*
C. Exotoxin of the *Clostridium tetani*
D. None of the above

19. Most common nerve involved in case of cephalic tetanus is:

A. Trigeminal nerve
B. Facial nerve
C. Trochlear nerve
D. Spinal accessory nerve

20. Metastatic stage of syphilis develops:

A. About six weeks after the primary lesion
B. About three weeks after contact with infection
C. About nine weeks after contact with infection
D. Several years after contact with infection

21. Which of the following stages of syphilis is/are noninfectious?

A. Primary stage B. Secondary stage
C. Tertiary stage D. All of the above

22. Secondary stage of syphilis characterized by:

A. Chancre B. Mucous patches
C. Syphilitic gumma D. Cardiovascular lesions

23. Herxheimer reaction is seen in:

A. Tuberculosis B. Syphilis
C. Sarcoidosis D. Herpetic gingivostomatitis

24. Intraoral gumma most commonly involves:

A. Gingiva B. Floor of mouth
C. Buccal mucosa D. Palate

25. Higoumenakis's sign is:

A. Hypoplasia of incisors and molars, eighth nerve deafness and interstitial keratitis
B. Rhagades and saber shin
C. Irregular thickening of the sternoclavicular portion of the clavicle
D. Saddle nose and short maxilla

26. Pseudobubo is seen in case of:

A. Lymphogranuloma venereum
B. Rhinoscleroma
C. Gonorrhea
D. Granuloma Inguinale

27. Which of the following is not a type of Donovanosis?

A. Cystic B. Ulcerative
C. Exuberant D. Cicatricial

28. Donovan bodies are present in:

A. Intracytoplasmic cyst within neutrophil
B. Cytoplasm of basophil
C. Intracytoplasmic cyst within eosinophil
D. Intracytoplasmic cyst within phagocytes

29. "Hebra nose" is seen in:

A. Granuloma venerum B. Gonorrhea
C. Scleroma D. Wegener's granulomatosis

30. Which of the following diseases does not appear clinically as midline lethal granuloma?

A. Sarcoidosis B. Brucellosis
C. Leishmaniasis D. Rhinoscleroma

31. Which of the followings causes Wegener's granulomatosis?

A. Chlamydia trachomatis
B. Klebsiella rhinoscleromatis
C. Calymmatobacterium granulomatis
D. None of the above

32. Mumps is caused by:

A. Orthomyxovirus B. Paramyxovirus
C. Rhabdovirus D. Retrovirus

33. Which of the followings is not a RNA virus?

A. Papovavirus B. Rhabdovirus
C. Picornavirus D. Togavirus

34. Herpes simplex is caused by:

A. RNA virus B. DNA virus
C. Retrovirus D. Pox virus

35. Herpes simplex virus type I causes infection in:

A. Skin of upper body
B. Skin of lower body
C. Genitals
D. None of the above

36. Herpes simplex virus type 2 remains latent in:

A. Ganglia of trigeminal nerve
B. Ganglia of lumbosacral region
C. Ganglia of thoracolumbar region
D. Ganglia of facial nerve

37. Lipschutz bodies are found in:

A. Herpes simplex virus infection
B. Syphilis
C. Aphthous ulcer
D. Herpangina

38. Which of the following is not included in classical triad of Behcet's syndrome?

A. Recurrent oral ulcer B. Recurrent skin ulcer
C. Recurrent genital ulcer D. Ocular inflammation

39. All of the following are included in tetrad of Reiter's syndrome *except*:

A. Conjunctivitis B. Arthritis
C. Urethritis D. None of the above

40. Reiter's syndrome is caused by:

A. Coxsackie group A virus
B. Pleuropneumonia-like organism
C. Herpes virus
D. Retrovirus

41. Acute lymphonodular pharyngitis is caused by:

A. Coxsackie virus A-15
B. Coxsackie virus A-10
C. Coxsackie virus A-12
D. Coxsackie virus A-5 and A-6

42. Hand, foot and mouth disease in caused by:

A. Coxsackie virus A-10
B. Coxsackie virus A-15
C. Coxsackie virus A-12
D. Coxsackie virus A-16

43. Variola is another name of:

A. Smallpox B. Morbilli
C. German measles D. Chickenpox

44. Henderson-Paterson inclusions are found in:

A. Chickenpox
B. Smallpox
C. Molluscum contagiosum
D Morbilli

45. Koplik's spots are found in:

A. Rubella B. Morbilli
C. Variola D. Varicella

46. Which of the following is wrong statement?

A. Herpes zoster is caused by reactivation of latent herpes simplex virus
B. It is typically unilateral or dermatomic in distribution
C. It involves face by infection of trigeminal nerve
D. Herpes zoster and herpes simplex can be differentiated by fluorescent antibody staining techniques

47. Which of the followings does not cause parotid swelling?

A. Sarcoidosis B. Malnutrition
C. Congenital atresia D. None of the above

48. Darling's disease is also known as:

A. Infectious mononucleosis B. Coccidioidomycosis
C. Histoplasmosis D. Lutz's disease

49. Kissing disease is another name of:

A. Histoplasmosis B. Coccidioidomycosis
C. Kimura's disease D. Glandular fever

50. Most opportunistic infection in the world is:

A. Leukoplakia
B. Tuberculosis
C. Herpetic gingivostomatitis
D. Candidiasis

51. Which of the following is also known as denture sore mouth?

A. Acute pseudomembranous oral candidiasis
B. Acute atrophic oral candidiasis
C. Chronic hyperplastic oral candidiasis
D. Chronic atrophic oral candidiasis

52. Which of the following looks like an oral leukoplakia?

A. Chronic diffuse mucocutaneous candidiasis
B. Chronic atrophic oral candidiasis
C. Chronic hyperplastic oral candidiasis
D. Chronic localized mucocutaneous candidiasis

53. In which of the following diseases chancres are found?

A. Rhinosporidiosis
B. Mucormycosis
C. Sporotrichosis
D. Geotrichosis

54. Oral thrush is also known as:

A. Acute atrophic oral candidiasis
B. Acute pseudomembranous oral candidiasis
C. Chronic atrophic oral candidiasis
D. Chronic hyperplastic oral candidiasis

Explanations

1.C. Scarlet fever, a disease that occurs predominantly in children during the winter months, is caused by infection with streptococcal organisms of the beta-hemolytic type that elaborate an erythrogenic toxin.

2.D. There is an incubation period of three to five days, after which the patient exhibits servere pharyngitis and tonsillitis, headache, chills, fever and vomiting.

3.C. Early in the course of disease, tongue exhibits a white coating, and the fungiform papillae are edematous and hyperemic, projecting above the surface as small red knobs. This phenomenon is clinically described as 'strawberry' tongue.

4.B. Rash, which is prominent in the areas of skin folds is a result of toxic injury to the vascular endothelium which produces dilatation of the small blood vessels and consequent hyperemia.

5.C. Diphtheria is an acute contagious disease caused by a gram-positive bacillus, cornybacterium diphthriae, or Klebs-Löffler bacillus.

6.C. There are no available methods for the prevention of scarlet fever.

7.A. Lesion may occur at any site on the oral mucous membrane, but the tongue is most commonly affected followed by the palate, lips, buccal mucosa, gingiva and frenule.

8.B. This specific form of tuberculosis probably arises as a resul of lymphatic spread of organisms from a focus of infection in the oral cavity such as the tonsils.

9.D. This disease has unknown etiology.

10.B. An intracutaneous test for the diagnosis of sarcoidosis, the Kveim-Siltzbach test, has been devised, utilizing a suspension of human known sarcoidal tissue as the test agent.

11.C. Heerfordt's syndrome is also known as uveoparotid fever.

12.B. Leprosy is a chronic granulomatous, infection caused by acid-fast bacillus, mycobacterium leprae.

13.D. A. bovis produces lumpy jaw in cattle but is seldom found to be a pathogen in humans.

14.B. If the pus from abscesses is carefully examined on a clean glass slide, it shows the typical "sulfur granules" or colonies of organisms which appear in the suppurative material as tiny yellow grains.

15.A. Trauma seems to play a role in some cases by initiating a portal of entry for the organisms, since they are not highly invasive.

16.B. Rabbit fever is also known as Tularemia.

17.B. After a variable incubation period of up to seven days, the patient usually suffers a sudden heodache, nausea, vomiting, chills and fever. A single cut or sore on the skin develop into ulcer. Lymph nodes become enlarged and painful.

18.C. Tetanus or lockjaw is caused by the exotoxin of the anaerobic gram- positive bacillus *Clostridium tetani.*

19.B. Cephalic tetanus is tetanus which is either localized or generalized, occurring in association with cranial nerve palsy, most commonly the seventh cranial nerve.

20.A. The second or metastatic stage, usually commencing about six weeks after the primary lesion is characterized by diffuse eruptions of skin and mucous membrane.

21.C. Tertiary syphilis, also called late syphilis, do not usually appear for several years and involve chiefly the cardio-vascular system, the central nervous system and certain other tissues and organs.

22.B. Mucous patches are usually multiple, painless, grayish-white plaques overlying an ulcerated surface.

23.B. The lesion appears as a firm nodular mass in the tissue which may subsequently ulcerate. Such an occurrence frequently follows vigorous antibiotic therapy, a herxheimer reaction.

24.D. Intraoral gumma most commonly involves the tongue and palate.

25.C. Higoumenaki's sign is thickening of the strernoclanicular portion of the clanicle.

26.D. Inguinal ulceration arises initially as a fluctuant swelling known as pseudobubo.

27.A. The varied clinical appearance of the lesion is the basis of classification i.e ulcerative, exuberant and cicatricial.

28.D. Donovan bodies are tiny, elongated basophilic and argyrophilic rods and present in profuse numbers within the macrophages.

29.C. The proliferative nasal masses may produce the configuration known as the Hebra nose.

30.A. The lethal granuloma is a most unusual condition described as an idiopathic progressive destruction of the nose, paranasal sinuses, palate, face and pharynx.

31.D. Wegener's granulomatosis is a disease of unknown etiology which basically involves the vascular, renal and respiratory systems. It is thought to be a hypersensitivity reaction to an unknown antigen.

32.B. Paramyxovirus also causes measles virus.

33.A. Papovavirus is a DNA virus.

34.B. Herpes simplex is caused by herpes virus, which is a DNA virus.

35.A. HSV type 1 usually affects the face, lips, oral cavity and upper body skin.

36.B. Herpes simplex virus type 1 remain latent in trigeminal gauglion.

37.A. Lipschutz bodies are eosinphilic, ovoid, homogenous structures within the nucleus which tend to displace the nucleolus and nuclear chomatin peripherally.

38.B. In Behcet's syndrome, at least two of the classic triad of the disease must be present: recurrent oral ulcers, recurrent gential ulcers and ocular inflammation.

39.D. Tetrad of reiter's syndrome include urethritis, arthritis, conjunctivitis and mucocutaneous lesions.

40.B. Reiter's syndrome is almost totally confined to men, usually 20 to 30 years of age.

41.B. Acute lymphonodular pharyngitis is an acute febritle disease caused by a strain of coxsackie virus A-10.

42.D. Hand, foot and mouth disease is an epidemic infection caused by the entero virus coxsackie A-16.

43.A. Smallpox is an acute viral disease which before the discovery of vaccination by Jenner, was epidemic in nature.

44.C. Henderson Peterson inclusion are large eosinophilic intracytoplasmic inclusion badies, also known as molluscum bodies.

45.B. Morbilli is another name of measles.

46.A. Herpes zoster is caused by reactivation of the latent V-Z virus, which had been acquired during a previous attack of chickenpox.

47.D. Different causes of parotid swelling include neoplastic, inflammatory, hypersensitivity and drug reaction, metabolic and miscellaneous.

48.C. Histoplasmosis is a generalized fungus infection caused by the organism histoplasma capsulatum.

49.D. Glandular fever is also known as infections mononualeosis.

50.D. Candidiasis is also known as moniliasis or oral thrush.

51.D. Denture sore mouth is diffuse inflammation of the denture –bearing area, often occurring with angular cheilitis.

52.C. The oral lesions consist of firm, white persistant plaques, usually on the lips, tongue and cheeks.

53.C. The skin lesion, often described as sporotrichotic "chancres" appear at the site of inoculation as firm red to purple nodules which soon ulceretc.

54.B. The oral lesions are characterized by the appearance of soft, white slightly elevated plaques most frequently occurring on the buccal mucosa and tongue, but also seen on the palate, gingival and floor of mouth.

7

Dental Caries

1. Average pH of plaque in caries-free person is:

A. 5.5 B. 6.5
C. 6.1 D. 7.1

2. How much percentage of organic matter is present in enamel?

A. 0.66% B. 0.76%
C. 0.56% D. 0.46%

3. Highest content of iodine is found in:

A. Enamel B. Dentin
C. Cementum D. Bone

Note= If asked about highest concentration then Ans. (C) is correct.

4. In pit and fissure caries of occlusal surface, apex of the cone-shaped carious lesion is present towards:

A. Dentinoenamel junction
B. Buccal surface of tooth
C. Occlusal surface of tooth
D. Lingual surface of tooth

Note= If asked about base then Ans. (A) is correct.

5. In smooth surface caries of the proximal surface base of the cone-shaped carious lesion is present towards:

A. Dentinoenamel junction
B. Occlusal surface
C. Lingual surface
D. Mesial surface

Note= If asked about apex then Ans. (A) is correct.

6. **Pore volume of sound enamel is:**
   A. 0.01% B. 1.0%
   C. 0.1% D. 0.001%

7. **Greatest demineralization of enamel in caries is found in:**
   A. Zone 1 B. Zone 2
   C. Zone 3 D. Zone 4

8. **In carious process the pioneer bacterias are present in:**
   A. Enamel lamellae B. Dentinal tubule
   C. Enamel tufts D. Peritubular dentin

9. **Miller's liquefaction foci are present in:**
   A. Candidiasis B. Leukoplakia
   C. Dental caries D. Tuberculosis

10. **Which of the following mechanisms is responsible for formation of Miller's liquefaction foci?**
    A. Focal coalescence and breakdown of enamel lamellae
    B. Focal coalescence and breakdown of enamel tufts
    C. Generalized breakdown of dentinal tubule
    D. Focal coalescence and breakdown of dentinal tubule

11. **Which of the following zones of carious dentin is known as zone of dentinal sclerosis?**
    A. Zone 1 B. Zone 2
    C. Zone 3 D. Zone 4

12. **What is the pH of plaque with extreme caries activity?**
    A. 6.6 B. 4.4
    C. 3.2 D. 5.1

Explanations

1.D. The pH of plaques in different persons varied, but averaged about 7.1in caries-free person to 5.5 in persons with extreme caries activity.

2.C. Enamel conrains approximately 0.56 percent organic matter, of which 0.18 percent is a type of keratin, 0.17 percent a soluble protein, possibly a glycoprotein, and the remainder citric acid and peptides.

3.D. Highest concentration of iodine is found in cementum.

4.C. Base of the cone-shaped carious lesion is present towards dentinoenamel junction.

5.D. Apex of the cone-shaped carious lesion is present towards dentinoenamel junction.

6.C. Zone 1 is slightly more porous than sound enamel, having a pore volume of 1 percent compared with 0.1 percent in sound enamel.

7.C. The body of the lesion lies between the relatively unaffected surface laryer and the dark zone.

8.B. In the earliest stages of caries when only a few tubules are involved, microarganisme may be found penetrating these tubules before there is any clinical evidence of the carious process. These have been termed "pioneer bacteria."

9.C. This 'focus' is an ovoid area of destruction, parallel to the course of the tubules and filled with necrotic debris which tends to increase in size by expansion.

10.D.

11.B. Zone 2 is zone of dentinal sclerosis characterized by deposition of calcium salts in dentinal tubules.

12.B.

8

Diseases of the Pulp and Periapical Tissues

1. The most frequent cause of pulpal inflammation is:

A. Bacteria
B. Trauma
C. Chemicals
D. Iatrogenic problems

2. Histologically, the dental pulp most closely resembles:

A. Nervous tissue
B. Vascular tissue
C. Granulation tissue
D. Loose connective tissue

3. The pathognomonic symptom of acute apical periodontitis is:

A. Sensitivity to heat
B. Tenderness on percussion
C. Intermittent pain
D. Widening of periodontal ligament

4. Radiographic evidence of osteogenesis in periapical lesions of average size requires:

A. 3-6 months
B. 6-12 months
C. 12-18 months
D. 1-2 years

5. An apical abscess and a periodontal abscess may be differentiated by:

A. Percussion test
B. Pulp vitality test
C. Radiographs
D. Palpation

6. The desired response in tooth with periapical lesion after endodontic therapy is:

A. Regeneration of alveolar bone
B. Deposition of apical cementum
C. Reestablishment of periodontal ligament
D. All of the above

7. **Symptoms of internal resorption include:**
   A. Constant unexplained toothache
   B. Pulpal discomfort in morning
   C. Completely symptom-free or mild pain at the tolerable level
   D. Throbbing pain

8. **Generalized malaise and elevated body temperature are frequently associated with:**
   A. Acute pulpitis
   B. Necrotic pulp
   C. Acute apical abscess
   D. Chronic apical periodontitis

9. **In periapical lesions, radiographs are of diagnostic importance because they show:**
   A. Size of lesion and distinguish between granuloma and cyst
   B. Extent of pulpal and periapical involvement
   C. Variation in density of structures
   D. Presence of an infection

10. **A granuloma, cyst and an abscess may be accurately distinguished by:**
    A. Pulp vitality test
    B. Radiographic examination
    C. Percussion
    D. Histologic examination

11. **Internal resorption is least likely to be seen in a tooth with:**
    A. Acute pulpitis
    B. Chronic pulpitis
    C. Necrotic pulp
    D. Apical periodontitis

12. **Internal resorption is treated by:**
    A. Pulpotomy
    B. Pulpectomy
    C. Extraction
    D. Pulp capping

13. **The primary response of pulp to tissue destruction is:**
    A. Calcification
    B. Inflammation
    C. Ulceration
    D. Mast cell degranulation

14. **The lesion associated with vital pulp is:**
    A. Periapical granuloma
    B. Periapical cyst
    C. Periapical abscess
    D. Condensing osteitis

15. A periapical cyst can be radiographically distinguished from a granuloma by injecting:

A. Polyacrylamide gel
B. Radiopaque dies
C. Iodine
D. Sodium chloride

16. Immediate treatment recommended for acute apical abscess is:

A. Incision and drainage
B. Prescribe antibiotics
C. Prescribe analgesics
D. No emergency treatment

17. Pulpitis occurring through blood-borne bacteria is called:

A. Retrograde pulpitis
B. Baro-odontalgia
C. Anachoretic pulpitis
D. None of the above

18. Condensing osteitis is most frequently seen in:

A. Maxillary incisor region
B. Mandibular first premolar area
C. Mandibular first molar area
D. Maxillary first molar area

19. Periapical cysts are most common in:

A. Maxillary anterior region
B. Mandibular anterior region
C. Maxillary premolar region
D. Mandibular molar region

20. Clinically, pulp polyp presents with:

A. Pain on percussion
B. Highly sensitive to touch
C. Asymptomatic tooth
D. All of the above

21. A chronic periapical abscess may be differentiated from periapical osteofibrosis by:

A. Pulp vitality tests
B. Radiographs
C. Percussion
D. Test cavity

22. In contrast to acute pulpitis, in chronic pulpitis threshold for stimulation by electric pulp tester is:

A. Increased
B. Decreased
C. Unaffected
D. May increase or decrease

23. The most common of all sequelae of pulpitis is:

A. Periapical granuloma B. Periapical cyst
C. Periapical abscess D. Apical cyst

24. The epithelialized lining in a periapical cyst is derived from:

A. Oral epithelium B. Epithelial rests of Malassez
C. Sulcular epithelium D. Antral mucosa

25. Periapical cyst is a:

A. True cyst B. False cyst
C. Fissural cyst D. Developmental cyst

26. Cholesterol crystals are found in:

A. Globulomaxillary cyst
B. Nasolabial cyst
C. Periapical cyst
D. Dentigerous cyst

27. The epithelial lining in pulp polyp is:

A. Stratified squamous B. Pseudostratified
C. Ciliated columnar D. Columnar

28. The epithelium lining of pulp polyp is derived from:

A. Epithelial rest of Malassez
B. Pulpal connective tissue
C. Antral mucosa
D. Oral epithelium

29. In treating a patient with a periapical abscess and a sinus tract, the sinus:

A. Is curetted out
B. Requires no special treatment
C. Persists throughout life
D. None of the above

30. Pulpal fibers associated with sharp, piercing pain are:

A. A-δ fibers B. C-fibers
C. E-fibers D. All of the above

31. A tooth sensitive to percussion indicates:

A. A necrotic pulp
B. A vital but inflamed pulp
C. Inflammation of apical periodontal ligament
D. Periapical cyst

32. In case of an acute periapical abscess, drainage should be preferably established through:

A. Extraoral incision
B. Bone tissue
C. Root canal
D. Any of the above

33. An acute exacerbation of a chromic abscess is called:

A. Pulpal abscess
B. Recurring abscess
C. Sterile abscess
D. Phoenix abscess

34. The dull, gnawing pain in pulp is associated with excitation of:

A. A-δ fiber
B. C-fibers
C. E-fibers
D. D-fibers

35. The result of pulp vitality test may be misleading:

A. When moist-gangrenous pulp is present in root canal
B. In multirooted teeth, when pulp in only one of the canals is necrotic
C. In extensive calcifications in pulp tissue
D. All of the above

36. In case of teeth with full coverage restoration, pulp vitality may be tested by:

A. Electric pulp test
B. Percussion
C. Carbon dioxide snow
D. Radiographs

37. Treatment of hyperemia includes:

A. Pulpotomy
B. Pulpectomy
C. Pulp capping
D. Removal of the etiological factor

38. 'Adenomatoid odontogenic tumour' is commonly associated with:

A. Unerupted tooth
B. Root resolved deciduous teeth.
C. Non-vital permanent tooth
D. Trauma

39. 'Dentigerous cyst' may be differentiated from 'adenomatoid odontogenic tumour' as former is commonly associated with:

A. Apical region of tooth
B. Unerupted third molar
C. Unerupted incisors or premolars
D. Both cannot be differentiated radiographically

40. All are true, *except*:

A. Radiolucency associated with unerupted third molar is most probably Klestadt's cyst
B. Solitary bone cysts lack epithelial lining
C. Adenoameloblastoma is more common in anterior maxilla
D. Cherubism commonly involves the mandible than the maxilla

41. The most common site of mandibular fracture is the:

A. Body
B. Symphysis
C. Angle
D. Condyle

42. 'Osteogenesis tarda' is also known as:

A. Lobestein type osteogenesis imperfecta
B. Autosomal dominant disorder
C. More severe form of osteogenesis imperfecta
D. All are true

43. Which of the following has the greater chance of malignant transformation?

A. Cherubism
B. Osteogenesis imperfecta
C. Paget's disease
D. Osteomalacia

44. The most common cause of ankylosis of TMJ is?

A. Osteoarthritis
B. Traumatic occlusion
C. Congenital syphilis
D. Trauma

45. All of the following are features of Gardner's syndrome *except*:

A. Osteomas
B. Unerupted supernumerary teeth
C. Osteosarcoma
D. Cutaneous sebaceous cysts

46. Multiple unerupted supernumerary teeth are seen in:

A. Craniofacial dysostosis
B. Cleidocranial dysplasia
C. Treacher Collins syndrome
D. Pierre Robin syndrome

47. 'Albright's syndrome' is associated with:

A. Paget's disease
B. Eosinophilic granuloma
C. Polystotic fibrous dysplasia
D. Monostotic fibrous dysplasia

48. Hyperparathyroidism causes:

A. Hypercementosis
B. Osteitis deformans
C. Osteogenesis imperfecta
D. Osteitis fibrosa cystica.

49. 'Ghost cells' are seen in:

A. Regional odontodysplasia
B. Calcifying odontogenic cyst
C. Calcifying odontogenic epidermal tumour
D. All of the above

50. 'Cervical burn out' is seen in periapical and bite wing view of:

A. Root Caries in molars
B. Intact proximal root surface of premolars
C. Hypercementosis
D. Cervical abrasions

51. 'Disinfectant' used for infection control during radiography is/are:

A. Iodophors
B. Chlorines
C. Phenols
D. All of the above

Explanations

1.A. Most cases of pulpitis are primarily a result of dental caries in which bacterial invasion of the dentin and pulp tissue occurs.

2.D. The dental pulp is a delicate connective tissue liberally interspersed with tiny blood vessels, lymphatics, myelinated and unmyelinated nerves, and undifferentiated connective tissue cells.

3.B. The first evidence that infection has spread beyond the confines of the tooth pulp may be a noticeable sensitivity of the involved tooth to percussion, or mild pain occasioned when biting or chewing on solid food.

4.B.

5.B. In case of a periapical abscess, the tooth will be non-viatal on pulp vitality test and in case of a periodontal abscess, it may or may not be vital.

6.D.

7.C. The evidence of the lesion may be the appearance of a pink hue on the crown of the tooth, which represents the hyperplastic, vascular pulp tissue filling the resorbed area and showing through the remaining overlying tooth substance.

8.C. Rapid extension to adjacent bone marrow spaces frequently occurs, producing an actual osteomyelitis.

9.C.

10.D. The apical periodontal cyst is histologically identical with the periapical granuloma, from which it is actually derived, except for the presence of the epithelium-lined lumen.

11.C. The cause of the pulpal inflammation and subsequent resorption of tooth substance is unknown, although an obvious carious exposure and accompanying pulp infection are sometimes present.

12.B. Once perforation of the crown or root has occurred, the tooth must usually be extracted.

13.B.

14.D. Condensing osteitis is an unusual reaction of bone to infection, occurring in instances of extremely high tissue resistance or in cases of a low-grade infection.

15.A. The apical periodontal cyst exhibits a thin, radiopaque line around the periphery of the radiolucent area, and this indicates a reaction of bone to slowly expanding mass.

16.A. This can be accomplished by either opening the pulp chamber or extracting the tooth.

17.C. Bacteria circulating in the blood stream tend to settle out or accumulate at sites of pulpal inflammation such as that which might follow some chemical or mechanical injury to the pulp.

18.C. Condensing osteitis is an unusal reaction of bone to infection, occurring in instances of extremely high tissue resistance or in cases of low- grade infection.

19.A. Periapical cyst is a common but not inevitable sequela of periapical granuloma originating as a result of bacterial infection and necrosis of dental pulp, nearly always following carious involvement of the tooth.

20.C. Because the hyperplastic tissue contains few nerves, it is relatively insensitive to manipulation.

21.A.

22.A. In electric pulp testing the objective is to stimulate a pulpal response by subjecting the tooth to an increasing degree of electric current.

23.A. In case of chromic periapical abscess, the pulp will test non-vital.

24.B. Periapical cyst presupposes physical, chemical or bacterial injury resulting in death of the pulp, followed by stimulation of the epithelial rests of Malassez, which are normally present in the periodontal ligament.

25.A. It is a true cyst, since the lesion consists of a pathologic cavity that is lined by epithelium and is often fluid filled.

26.C. This mass of cholesterol frequently erodes through the lining epithelium and is extruded into the cyst lumen.

27.A. The epithelium is stratified squamous in type and closely resembles the oral mucosa, even to the extent of developing well formed rete pegs.

28.D. The grafted epithelial cells are thought to be normally desquamated cells carried to the surface of the pulp by the saliva.

29.B. Incision and drainage is the treatment for periapical abscess.

30.A. Sharp, piercing, lancinating pain in a tooth usually responds prompily to cold and is easy to localize.

31.C. This test helps to corroborate the presence of periodontitis.

32.C. Treatment consists of establishing drainage and controlling the systemic reaction. When symptoms have subsided, the tooth should be treated endodontically by conservative means.

33.D. Phoenix abscess is an acute inflammatory reaction superimposed on an existing chronic lesion, such as a cyst or granuloma.

34.B. Inability to localize the pain frequently relates to dental pain that is dull, boring and gnawing, from a tooth that responds abnormally to heat more than to cold.

35.D. Cause for confusion in multirooted teeth occur when the pulp is partially necrotic, with some nerve fibers still vital in one or more of the root canals.

36.C. Electric pulp testing is not done on teeth with full coverage restorations because an electrical stimulus cannot pass undistorted through acrylic, ceramic or metallic portiors of a crown.

37.D. Hyperemia is also known as acute reversible pulpitis.

38.A. The tumor is associated with an unerupted tooth and in over two-thirds of the cases, this tooth is maxillary or mandibular cuspid.

39.B. The adematoid odontogenic tumor is associated with an unerupted tooth in the anterior region.

40.A. Radiolucency associated with unerupted third molar is most probably dentigerous cyst.

41.C. This is due to the thinness of bone and difference in direction of grains.

42.D. Osteogenesis imperfecta when arise during childhood, it is known as tarda or Lobstein's type.

43.C. The most serious complication of Paget's disease is the development of osteosarcoma in a significant percentage of cases.

44.D. The most frequent causes of ankylosis of TMJ are traumatic injuries and infections in and about the joint.

45.C. Other features include desmoid tumors and multiple polyposis of large intestine.

46.B. Cleidoccranial dysplasia is also known as Marie and Sainton's disease.

47.C. Polyostotic fibrous dysplasia as severe as that in Albright's syndrome is a relatively uncommon disease and is marked by the presence of endocrinal disorders.

48.D. Hyperparathyroidism is a disease in which the parathyroid glands elaborate an ecessive quantity of parathyroid hormone.

49.D. Ghost cells are pale, eosinophilic, swollen epithelial cells that have lost the nucleus but show a faint outline of the cellular and nuclear membrane.

50.B.

51.D.

9

Spread of Oral Infection

1. Spreading factor of Duran-Reynals is also known as:

A. Hyaluronic acid
B. Chondroitin sulfate
C. Fibrinolysinase
D. Hyaluronidase

2. Cellulitis in head and neck region is caused by:

A. Dental infection
B. Pericoronal infection
C. Infection following a tooth extraction
D. All of the above

3. Which of the followings is not a correct statement?

A. In case of true Ludwing's angina all submandibular spaces are involved
B. Chondroitin sulfate is universal intercellular substance
C. Most commonly involved teeth in case of Ludwig's angina are second and third molars
D. Most cases of Ludwing's angina are a mixed infection

4. Infection from face and lip goes to cavernous sinus through:

A. Facial vein
B. Angular vein
C. Both of the above
D. Pterygoid plexus

5. Which of the following infections must always be considered in cases of acute or chronic maxillary sinusitis especially in diabetic cases?

A. Phycomycosis
B. Sporotrichosis
C. Coccidioidomycosis
D. Cryptococcosis

6. "Sinus Polyps" are present in:

A. Acute maxillary sinusitis
B. Chronic maxillary sinusitis
C. Ludwig's angina
D. Cellulitis

7. Infection in submasseteric space usually occurs from:

A. Mandibular first molar
B. Mandibular second molar
C. Mandibular third molar
D. Maxillary third molar

8. Phlegmon is also known as:

A. Cellulitis
B. Acute periapical abscess
C. Chronic periapical abscess
D. Ludwig's angina

9. Which of the following muscles is responsible for swelling in upper half of face in case of infection arising in maxilla?

A. Zygomaticus major
B. Zygomaticus minor
C. Buccinator
D. Risorious

10. Which of the followings is not included in infratemporal space?

A. Pterygoid plexus
B. External pterygoid muscle
C. Internal pterygoid muscle
D. Buccinator nerve

11. Which of the following spaces is not included in true Ludwig's angina?

A. Submandibular
B. Pterygomandibular space
C. Submental
D. Sublingual

Explanations

1.D. Hyaluronidase (the spreading factor of Duran – Reynals) act to break down or dissolve hyaluronic acid, the universal intercellular cement substance.

2.D. Sometimes cellulitis of the face or neck will occur as a result of injection with an infected needle or through an infected area, or following jaw fracture.

3.B. Chandroitin sulfate is connective tissue substance most commonly present in cornea and cartilage. Most cases of Ludwig's angina are a mixed infection, but Streptococci are almost invariably present.

4.C. Infection from the face and lip is carried by the facial and angular vein, while dental infection is carried by way of the pterygoid plexus.

5.A. Phycomycosis is a fungul disease. Early clinical manifestation of the disease is the appearance of a reddish-black nasal turbinate and septum with a nasal discharge.

6.B. Sinus polyps are simple hyperplastic granulation tissue with lymphocytic and sometimes plasma cell infiltration.

7.C. Submassetric space infection usually occurs from a mandible third molar, the infection passing through the retromolar fossa and into the submassetric space.

8.A. Cellulitis is a diffuse inflammation of soft tissues which is not circumscribed or confined to one area, but which, in contradistinction to the abscess, tends to spread through tissue spaces and along fascial planes.

9.C. When infection in the mandible perforates the outer contical plate below the buccinator attachment there is a diffuse swelling of the lower half of the face which then spreads superiorly as well as cervically.

10.C. The infratemporal space contains the pterygoid plexus, the internal maxillary artery, the mandibular, mylohyoid, lingual, buccinator and chorda tympani nerves and the external pterygoid muscle.

11.B. Ludwig's angina is a severe cellulites beginning usually in the submaxillary space and secondarily involving the sublingual and submental spaces as well.

10

Physical and Chemical Injuries of the Oral Cavity

1. Which of the followings is least injurious to the tooth?

A. $Ca(OH)_2$ B. ZOE (Zinc oxide eugenol)
C. Zinc phosphate D. Composite resin

2. What is the remaining thickness of primary dentin over which a cement base is necessary?

A. 2.0 cm B. 0.2 mm
C. 0.02 mm D. Less than 2.0 mm

3. According to Ellis classification of traumatized teeth, teeth lost as a result of trauma is:

A. Class IV B. Class V
C. Class VI D. Class VII

4. All of the following are true about tooth ankylosis *except*:

A. Deciduous teeth ankylosis is not known as submerged teeth
B. Tooth ankylosis is common in deciduous teeth than permanent teeth
C. On percussion there is dull muffled sound
D. Periodontal ligament is completely obliterated in area of ankylosis

5. Which of the following is not a traumatic bone cyst?

A. Static bone cyst B. Hemorrhagic cyst
C. Extravasation cyst D. Unicameral bone cyst

6. Pathomimia mucosae oris is:

A. Cheek biting B. Lip biting
C. Biting habits D. Sore spots

7. **Denture injury tumor is:**
   A. Denture sore mouth
   B. Sore spots
   C. Epulis fissuratum
   D. Palatal papillomatosis

8. **Mucous retention phenomena are usually found in:**
   A. Upper lip
   B. Lower lip
   C. Floor of mouth
   D. Gingiva

9. **Which of the following is a true cyst?**
   A. Static bone cyst
   B. Haemorrhagic bone cyst
   C. Extravasation cyst
   D. None of the above

10. **Sialolithiasis is most common in:**
    A. Parotid gland duct
    B. Submandibular gland duct
    C. Sublingual gland duct
    D. Accessory salivary gland duct

11. **Highest content of salivary duct stone is made up of:**
    A. $CaCO_3$
    B. $Ca_3(PO_4)_2$
    C. Soluble salts
    D. Water

12. **Bismuth was primarily used in treatment of:**
    A. Epilepsy
    B. Tuberculosis
    C. Syphilis
    D. Morsus humanus

13. **"Test-tube" pegs are found in:**
    A. Lichen planus
    B. Candidiasis
    C. Dilantin sodium induced fibrous hyperplasia
    D. Mercury poisoning

14. **Which of the following is common in acute mercurial poisoning but does not occur in chronic mercurial poisoning?**
    A. Tremors of fingers
    B. Desquamative dermatitis
    C. Nephritis
    D. Insomnia

15. **Pink disease occurs due to poisoning of:**
    A. Bismuth
    B. Lead
    C. Mercury
    D. Iron

16. Which of the following does not occur in mercury poisoning?

A. Metallic taste in mouth
B. Increased flow of saliva
C. Decreased flow of saliva
D. Swelling in salivary gland

17. Argyria is due to poisoning of:

A. Mercury B. Silver
C. Gold D. Copper

18. Which of the following is absent in hereditary form of Quinke's edema?

A. C′ 2 esterase inhibitor B. C′1 esterase inhibitor
C. C′3 esterase inhibitor D. C′4 esterase inhibitor

19. All of the following are radioresistant *except*:

A. Pancreas B. Liver
C. Conjunctiva D. Pituitary

20. What is the upper limit of Roentgen for a radio responsive cell?

A. 2,500 Roentgen B. 5,000 Roentgen
C. 7,500 Roentgen D. 10,000 Roentgen

21. Burtonian line is associated with:

A. Bismuth B. Mercury
C. Lead D. Iron

22. Which of the following serve as an index of the body burden of lead?

A. Incisors B. Molars
C. Deciduous teeth D. Permanent teeth

23. Which of the following is not correct?

A. Lead poisoning is known as plumbism
B. Lead line is more clear than bismuth line
C. Gastrointestinal disturbances are common in bismuth poisoning
D. Bismuth line is blue or black in color

24. Wrist-drop develops due to peripheral neuritis in:

A. Mercury poisoning
B. Lead poisoning
C. Iron poisoning
D. Bismuth poisoning

Explanations

1.B. Zinc oxide and eugenol produces no irritation and exerts a palliative and sedative effect on the mildly damaged pulp.

2.D. If the cavity depth is shallow, with 2.0 mm or more of primary dentin remaining between the floor of the cavity preparation and the dental pulp, dentin probably provides its own insulation against traumatic, thermal or restorative material irritation. When it is less than 2 mm a cement base becomes necessary.

3.B. Boys are more frequently involved than girls. There is a definite predilection for involvement of maxillary teeth, with between 75 and 90 percent of fractures occurring there.

4.A. Ankylosis ensues when partial root resorption is followed by repair with either cementum or bone that unites the tooth root with the alveolar bone.

5.A. Solitary bone cyst, simple bonecyst and idiopathic bone cavity are also traumatic bone cyst.

6.C. Lip-biting is morsicatio labiorum and cheek biting is morsicatio buccarum.

7.C. Denture injury tumor is also known as inflammatory fibrous hyperplasia and occurs due to an ill fitting denture.

8.B. The retention phenomenon involving accessory salivary gland structures occurs most frequently on the lower lip, but may alos occur on the palate, cheek, tongue and floor of mouth.

9.D. All these are not true cyst. The term 'cyst' is actually a misnomer, since these intrabony cavities are not lined by epithelium.

10.B. The common involvement of the submaxillary gland and duct is thought to be due to the tenacity of the submaxillary saliva, which, because of its high mucin content, adheres to any foreign particle .The submaxillary duct is also long and irregular in its course.

11.B. Wakeley reported the average composition of apatite structure as follows.

$Ca_3(PO_4)_2$	74.3%
$CaCO_3$	11.1%
Soluble salts	6.2%
Organic matter	6.2%
Water	2.2%

12.C. Bismuth was formerly used widely in the treatment of syphilis, but it has been replaced in recent years by the antibiotics.

13.C. Test tube pegs are rete pegs, which are extremely long and thin.

14.C. Chronic mercurialism is characterized by gastric disturbances, diarrhea, excitability, insomnia, headache and mental depression. Patients frequently have fine tremors of fingers, limbs lips and tongue.

15.C. Pink disease is also known as acrodynia or Swift's disease.

16.C. Increased flow of saliva is also known as ptyalism.

17.B. Chronic exposure to silver compounds may occur as an occupational hazard or as the result of therapeutic use of silver compounds such as silver arsphenamine or silver nitrate.

18.B. In Quinck's disease, there is absence of normally naturally occurring inhibitor of CI estearase, which is a specific α-2 globulin in the complement system. This leads to increased consumption of C'^2 and C'^4, which in turn causes increased; kinin production thereby increased capillary permeability and edema.

19.C. Salivary glands, bone and cartilage, epithelium of blood vessels and collagen and elastic tissue are also radio-responsive.

20.B. Lower limit of Roentgen for a radio responsive cell is 2500 Roentgen.

21.C. Burtonian line is gray or bluish-black line of sulfide pigmentation .It occurs in the gingiva but is somewhat more diffuse than that of bismuth.

22.C. Lead is deposited in the deciduous teeth of children suffering from lead poisoning and that these teeth may serve as an index of the body burden of lead.

23.B. Lead intoxication is manifested by serious gastrointestinal disturbances, which include nausea, vomiting, colic and constipation. Lead line is present on the gingiva but is more diffuse.

24.B. A foot drop sign may also develop. Encephalitis may also occur. Blood changes are those of a hypochromic anemia with basophilic stippling of the red blood cells.

11

Healing of Oral Wounds

1. **Which of the following vitamins is not involved in healing of oral wounds?**

   A. Vit. D B. Pyridoxine
   C. Riboflavin D. Vit. E

2. **Biopsy used in follow-up detection of recurrent carcinoma in previously treated cases is:**

   A. Exfoliative cytology B. Incisional biopsy
   C. Excisional biopsy D. Pouch biopsy

3. **What is the class of cytologic smear which separates cancer from noncancer diagnosis?**

   A. Class II B. Class III
   C. Class IV D. Class V

4. **Which of the following classes of cytologic smear is suggestive of cancer?**

   A. Class III B. Class IV
   C. Class V D. Class II

5. **Organisation of blood clot occurs after:**

   A. One week B. Two weeks
   C. Two days D. Four days

6. **Epithelialization of gingivectomy wound is completed after:**

   A. Four days B. Two weeks
   C. Four weeks D. Two months

7. **After how many weeks of extraction radiographic evidence of healing becomes prominent?**

   A. Four weeks B. Six weeks
   C. Ten weeks D. Twelve weeks

8. Most common complication in the healing of human extraction wounds is:

A. Loss of blood clot
B. Generalized osteomyelitis
C. Alveolitis sicca dolorosa
D. Lack of organization of blood clot

9. Dry socket occurs most commonly with impacted:

A. Mandibular first molar B. Mandibular third molar
C. Maxillary first molar D. Maxillary canine

10. Dry socket generally develops after:

A. Two days of extraction
B. Four days of extraction
C. One week of extraction
D. Four hours of extraction

Explanations

1.D. Vitamin A deficiency retards healing and that vitamins A and D, as in cod liver oil, may be factors in promoting tissue repair. B complex vitamin deficiecy also retards wound heading.

2.A. Exfoliative cytology is a quick, simple, painless and bloodless procedure. It helps as a check against false negative biopsies.

3.B. The cells display wider atypia that may be suggestive of cancer, but they are not clear-cut and may represent precancerous lesions or carcinoma in situ.

4.B. A few cells with maligment characteristics or many cell with borderline characteristics.

5.D. Four days after the operation the deeper portion of the blood clot demonstrates considerable organization, while the more superficial portion exhibits dense numbers of polymorphonuclear leukocytes entrapped in the fibrinous meshwork.

6.B. Epithelialization is usually complete within ten to fourteen days after gingivectomy.

7.B. Roentgenographic evidence of bone formation does not become prominent untill the sixth or eighth week after tooth extraction.

8.C. Alveolitis sicca dolorosa is also known as dry socket.

9.B. The condition is most frequently associated with difficult or traumatic extractions and thus most commonly follows removal of an impacted mandibular third molar.

10.B. The dry socket is basically a focal osteomyelitis in which the blood clot has disintegrated or been lost, with the production of a foul odor and severe pain, but no suppuration.

12

Aspects of Metabolic Diseases

1. Which of the following can replace calcium in the inorganic structure of bone?

A. Rubidium
B. Lead
C. Selenium
D. Potassium

2. Serum calcium ion concentration is:

A. 19 to 21 mg/dl
B. 0.9 to 1.1 mg/dl
C. 9 to 11 mg/dl
D. 9 to 11 gm/dl

3. Which of the following do not occur in high concentration of calcium in blood?

A. Convulsions
B. Depressed nerve conductivity
C. Muscle rigor
D. None of the above

4. How much percentage of daily dietary intake of calcium is not absorbed under normal condition?

A. 33%
B. 45%
C. 75%
D. 67%

5. Which of the following can increase calcium absorption?

A. Phytic acid
B. High protein diet
C. Increase in intestinal pH
D. Low fat diet

6. Which of the following elements can replace potassium in a potassium-deficient diet?

A. Ruthenium
B. Rubidium
C. Lead
D. Strontium

7. All of the following are essential elements *except*:

A. Chromium
B. Strontium
C. Selenium
D. Zinc

8. Renal threshold for calcium is approximately:

A. 11 mg/dl of serum calcium
B. 7 mg/dl of serum calcium
C. 15 mg/dl of serum calcium
D. 9 mg/dl of serum calcium

9. Blood level of phosphate is maintained by:

A. Vitamin A
B. Phosphatase activity
C. Both of the above
D. Thyroid hormone

10. Which of the following enzymes activity depends on magnesium?

A. Phosphorylase
B. Phosphatase
C. Cocarboxylase
D. All of the above

11. At which serum magnesium level profound coma or death may occur?

A. 1-3 mg/dl
B. 3-5 mg/dl
C. 9-11 mg/dl
D. 18-21 mg/dl

12. Deposition of calcium salts in degenerating tissue is known as:

A. Dystrophic calcification
B. Metastatic calcification
C. Calcinosis
D. Tetany

13. Most common location of intraoral dystrophic calcification is:

A. Tongue
B. Cheek
C. Gingiva
D. Floor of mouth

14. Which of the following statements is not correct?

A. Nodular type of dystrophic calcification is common in radicular pulp of tooth
B. Normal serum magnesium level is 1 to 3 mg/dl
C. Calcinosis circumscripta is not associated with scleroderma
D. Calcinosis is presence of calcifications in or under the skin

15. How much percentage of sodium is present in enamel ash?

A. 3.0%
B. 0.3%
C. 0.03%
D. 0.003%

16. The normal blood level of sodium is:

A. 160 mg/dl of whole plasma
B. 340 mg/L of whole plasma
C. 310 mg/dl of whole plasma
D. 340 mg/dl of whole plasma

17. Most of sodium and potassium inside the body is:

A. Extracellular
B. Intracellular
C. Extracellular and intracellular respectively
D. Intracellular and extracellular respectively

18. Which of the following enzymes is activated by chloride ion?

A. Pancreatic lipase
B. Pancreatic amylase
C. Salivary amylase
D. Pepsin

19. How much of total body iodine is found in thyroid?

A. Half
B. One-third
C. Two-third
D. Almost all

20. Which of the following occurs due to copper deficiency?

A. Wilson's disease
B. Menkes syndrome
C. Both of the above
D. None of the above

21. Which of the following is a "one-way substance?"

A. Manganese
B. Copper
C. Magnesium
D. Iron

22. Which of the following can cause iron overload in body?

A. Sideroblastic anemia
B. Bantu siderosis
C. Both of the above
D. Steely-or Kinkyhair syndrome

23. Maximum concentration of zinc is found in:

A. Bone
B. Pancreas
C. Spleen
D. Dentin

24. What is the concentration of zinc in enamel?

A. 0.2%
B. 2.0%
C. 0.02%
D. 0.002%

25. Which of the following ions concentration in the teeth is found at higher level in tuberculosis?

A. Copper
B. Manganese
C. Cobalt
D. Zinc

26. Acrodermatitis enteropathica is associated with:

A. Copper
B. Zinc
C. Manganese
D. Magnesium

27. Which of the following ions is associated with activity of glutathione peroxidase?

A. Zinc
B. Chromium
C. Selenium
D. Fluoride

28. Which of the following is correct about protein requirement of the body?

A. 1 gm of protein per kg body weight
B. 1 gm of protein per gm body weight
C. 1 mg of protein per gm body weight
D. 1 mg of protein per kg body weight

29. Which of the following is not an essential amino acid?

A. Tryptophan
B. Tyrosine
C. Histidine
D. Threonine

30. Which of the following amino acids is essential for infants but nonessential for adults?

A. Histidine
B. Valine
C. Arginine
D. Leucine

31. Amyloid deposited in case of multiple myeloma is:

A. Type A
B. Type B
C. Type C
D. None of the above

32. All of the following include a subclass of hepatic porphyria *except*:

A. Porphyria variegata
B. Porphyria cutanea tarda
C. Protoporphyria
D. Hereditary coproporphyria

33. Under ultraviolet light, porphyric teeth show:

A. Green fluorescence
B. Yellow fluorescence
C. Orange fluorescence
D. Red fluorescence

34. Gargoylism is another name of:

A. Lipoid proteinosis
B. Histiocytosis X disease
C. Hurler syndrome
D. Histiocytosis Y disease

35. Reilly bodies are present in:

A. Histiocytosis X disease
B. Hyalinosis cutis et mucosae
C. Hand-Schüller-Christian disease
D. Mucopolysaccharidosis I

36. Inability of infants to cry at birth, is characteristic finding of:

A. Hurler syndrome B. Lipoid Proteinosis
C. Letterer-Siwe disease D. Gaucher's disease

37. All of the following are nonlipid reticuloendotheliosis *except*:

A. Letterer-Siwe disease
B. Eosinophilic granuloma
C. Niemann-Pick disease
D. Hand-Schüllar-Christian disease

38. Proliferative cell in multifocal eosinophilic granuloma is:

A. Eosinophil B. Neutrophil
C. Lymphocyte D. Histiocyte

39. All of the following are features of Letterer-Siwe disease *except*:

A. Diffuse skeletal involvement occurs only
B. It involves children usually before the age of three years
C. Foam cells are not a feature of this disease
D. Proliferating cells are histiocytes

40. In Gaucher's disease there is deposition of:

A. Sphingosine B. Kerasin
C. Chondroitin sulfate D. Hyaluronic acid

41. Gaucher's cells are:

A. Lipid filled lymphocyte B. Lipid filled neutrophil
C. Lipid filled eosinophil D. Lipid filled histiocyte

42. All of the following are correct about Niemann-Pick cell *except*:

A. Unlike Gaucher cell they are strongly positive for alkaline phosphatase
B. Unlike Gaucher cell they are positive for cholesterol
C. They are very easily distinguished from Gaucher cells by phase or electron microscopy
D. They are lipid laden cells

43. Disturbances in glucosyl ceramide metabolism is found in:

A. Gaucher's disease B. Niemann-Pick disease
C. Letterer-Siwe disease D. Hurler syndrome

44. 1-α-hydroxylase needed in vit D metabolism is found in

A. Hepatic tissue B. Kidney
C. Heart D. Lung

45. Vitamin D_2 is also known as

A. Cholecalciferol B. Ergosterol
C. 7-dehydrocholesterol D. Ergocalciferol

46. Which of the following is/are also known as phosphate diabetes?

A. Adult rickets B. Refractory rickets
C. Both of the above D. Renal rickets

47. All are correct about hypophosphatasia *except*:

A. Deficiency of alkaline phosphatase
B. Excretion of phosphopantothenic acid
C. Severity is not related to alkaline phosphatase level
D. Absence of cementum

48. Daily dietary intake of Vitamin C should be:

A. 60 mg in infants and 120 mg in adults
B. 120 mg in infants and 240 mg in adults
C. 35 mg in infants and 60 mg in adults
D. 15 mg in infants and 35 mg in adults

49. Trümmerfeld zone is associated with:

A. Vitamin E B. Vitamin C
C. Vitamin A D. Vitamin D

50. Pseudocyst formation occurs in:

A. Primary hyperparathyroidism
B. Secondary hyperparathyroidism
C. Hypothyroidism
D. Hyperthyroidism

Explanations

1.B. Strontium or lead may replace calcium in the inorganic structure of bone. Rubidium may replace potassium in a potassium-deficient diet.

2.C. A low concertration of calcium ions (about 8 mg/dl) produces hyperirritability and tetany with characteristic carpopedal spasm while a high concentration produces depressed nerve conductivity and muscle rigor.

3.A. The level of the blood calcium is largely controlled by the action of parathyroid glands, which are stimulated by low serum calcium levels and inhibited by high serum calcium levels.

4.D. The absorption of calcium in man is an inefficient process. Only about one-third of the daily dietary intake of calcium is absorbed under normal conditions.

5.B. High protein diets have been shown to increase calcium absorption, probably through the formation of soluble cacium compound with the amino acid produced by the digestion of the protein.

6.B. Even through the animals maintained on the diet die, the characteristic myocardial necrosis found in potassium deficiency will not occur.

7.B. The elements considered essential for normal growth and development of mammals are calcium, phosphorous, magnesium, potassium, sodium, chlorine, iodine, copper, iron, zinc, manganese, cobalt, chromium, selenium and fluoride.

8.B. The calcium in the urine is excreted mainly as calcium chloride and calcium phosphate.

9.B. Blood levels are maintained by a balance of various factors, such as parathyroid hormone, phosphatase activity and vitamin D.

10.D. Magnesium appears to participate in practically every phosphorylating mechanism. In addition, this ion is necessary for the activity of certain enzymes, such as phosphatase and cocarboxylase.

11.D. The normal serum magnesium level is 1 to 3 mg/dl.

12.A. Areas of tuberculous necrosis, blood vessels in arteriosclerosis, scars and areas of fatty degeneration are commonly recognized as sites of dystrophic calcification.

13.C. In the mouth, areas of dystrophic calcification may frequently be found in the gingiva, tongue or cheek.

14.A. Noclular type of dystrophic calcification is a result of calcification of hyalinized connective tissue. It is found in the coronal portion of pulp chamber.

15.B. The sodium ion content of the normal (70 kg) adult male ranges from 83 to 97 gm.

16.D. Normal blood level is 160 mg/dl of whole blood, or 340 mg/dl of plasma.

17.C. Most of the sodium is extracellular and accounts for 90 percent of the basic ions of both extracellular fluid and plasma.

18.C. Chlorine is one of the so-called threshold substance which are reabsorbed into the circulation after passing through the glomeruli to maintain normal body fluid concentrations.

19.B. Iodine is essential for the formation of thyroid hormone.

20.C. Human Cooper deficiency diseases of importance are hepatolenticular degeneration (Wilson's disease) and Menkes syndrome (steely or kinky hair syndrome).

21.D. Since little excretion of iron takes place either by the alimentary canal or by the kidneys, this element has been called a 'one way substance'.

22.C. Bantu siderosis, a form of iron overload results from ingestion of homemade beer fermented in iron pots.

23.D. The concentration of zinc in enamel and dentin is about 0.02 percent, which is higher than in any other tissue of the body.

24.C. Bone, nails and hair have slightly lower concentrations.

25.D. A strange and unexplained observation is that the teeth of tuberculous patients apparently have a higher zinc concentration than the teeth of normal people.

26.B. Its symptoms include diarrhea and a wide range of mucocutancous problems including vesicles, eczematoid and hyperkeratotic plaques, alopecia, stomatitis and glossitis.

27.C. Glutathione peroxidase is a selenoenzyme that is responsible for eliminating potentially harmful peroxides and free radicals.

28.A. Protein is required in increased quantity in the last half of pregnancy and during lactation and in even greater amount in infancy, childhood and adolescence.

29.B. The essential amino acids are histidine, isoleucine, leucine, lysine, methionine, phenylalanine, threonine, tryptophan and valine.

30.C. Infants are incapable of producing sufficient amounts of arginine for normal psysiologic function. Therefore, arginine is considered essential in infants.

31.B. Type B amyloid is commonly seen in patients with multiple myelome and macroglobulinemia.

32.C. Hepatic porphyria is a multisystem disorder, which has four subclasses–acute intermittent porphyria, prophyria veriegata, prophyria cutanea tarda and hereditary coproporphyria.

33.D. Prophyria is a term which has been generally used to connote one of the inborn errors of porphyrin metabolism, characterized by overproduction of uroporphyrin and related substances.

34.C. Hurler syndrome is a syndrome of mucopolysacchand metabolism characterized by an elevated mucopolysaccharide excretion level in the urine.

35.D. Metachromatic granules or Reilly bodies can often be demonstrated in the cytoplasm of circulating lymphocytes.

36.B. Lipoid proteinosis is a disease characterized by disturbance in mucopolysaccharide metabolism, or an alteration involving lipoprotein material.

37.C. Non lipid reticuloendothelioses is also known as histiocytosis X disease.

38.D. Hand-Schuller-Christian disease, Letterer-Siwe disease and eosinophilic granuloma of bone have traditionally been grouped under the generic term histiocytosis X and the proliferative cell is the histiocyte.

39.A. Histiocytes do not contain significant amounts of cholesterol so that foam cells are not a feature of the disease, nor is fibrosis encountered.

40.B. Gaucher's disease is an autosomal receissive defect of lipid metabolism in which kerasin is deposited throughout the entire reticuloendothelial system as a result of a deficiency in glucocerebrosidase.

41.D. Gaucher's disease has been divided into three clinical forms (type I, II, and III,).

42.A. Niemann-pick cells are foamy, lipid laden cells distributed throughout the reticuloendothelial system.

43.B.

44.B. Renal rickets results from the inability of diseased kidneys to synthesize 1-α-hydroxylase and convert 25-hydroxychole calciferol to the active form of vitamin D i.e. 1,25 dihydroxycholecalciferol (CALCITRIOL)

45.D. Vitamin D_3 is also known as cholecalciferol.

46.B. Refractory rickets is also known as vitamin D-Resistant rickets.

47.B. Absence of cementum occurs as a result of cementogenesis, so that there is no sound functional attachment of the tooth to bone by periodontal ligament.

48.C. Pregnant and lactating women should increase their daily intake by 20 mg and 40 mg respectively.

49.B. Fracturing of the calcified matrix material leads to the classic picture of scurvy, the so called trummerfeldzone or region of complete disintegration.

50.A. Extent of pseudocyst formation depends on the duration and intensity of the disease.

13

Oral Aspects of Metabolic Disease

1. Lamina dura around the teeth may be partially lost in:

A. Ehlers-Danlos syndrome
B. Secondary hyperparathyroidism
C. Primary hyperparathyroidism
D. Osteosarcoma

2. "Brown's tumors" are associated with:

A. Primary hyperparathyroidism
B. Secondary hyperparathyroidism
C. Hyperthyroidism
D. Hypothyroidism

3. Coxa valga is a constant feature of:

A. Hutchinson-Gilford syndrome
B. Hurler syndrome
C. Both of the above
D. Marfan-Achard syndrome

4. Children who do not drink milk are deficient in:

A. Vitamin A
B. Riboflavin
C. Pantothenic acid
D. Thiamine

5. Gerustmark is associated with deficiency of:

A. Vitamin B complex
B. Vitamin D
C. Vitamin A
D. Vitamin C

6. Pellagra is due to deficiency of:

A. Vitamin B1
B. Vitamin B2
C. Niacin
D. Nicotinic acid

Explanations

1.C. In the jaws, the bone roentgenogram in hyperparathyroidism has been described as having a ground glass appearance.

2.B. Loss of lamina dura is also a prominent finding.

3.A.

4.B. Riboflavin (vitamin B_2) is a fully dialyzable, intensely yellow water-soluble pigment, which is decomposed by light.

5.D. The area beneath the trummerfeldzone is free of hematopoietic cells and is made up of connective tissue cells, the so called gerustmark.

6.C. The world pellagra means rough skin.

14

Diseases of Bone and Joints

1. "Brittle bones" is also known as:

A. Osteoporosis B. Osteogenesis imperfecta
C. Osteopsathyrosis D. Both (B) and (C)

2. The form of osteogenesis imperfecta present in childhood is known as:

A. Congenita type B. Vrolik's type
C. Both of the above D. Gravis type

3. All of the following are characteristic of Lobestein's disease *except*:

A. Extreme fragility and porosity of the bones
B. On the fracture site new bone of similar imperfect quality is formed
C. Sometimes hypoplastic callus formation occurs on fracture site
D. Sarcoma can develop into the lesion

4. Blue sclera is found in:

A. Ehlers-Danlos syndrome B. Fetal rickets
C. Fragilitas ossium D. All of the above

5. Basic defect in Lobestein's disease is:

A. Failure in maturation of bone
B. Failure in calcification of bone
C. Failure in maturation of collagen fibers
D. All of the above

6. In which of the following conditions white sclerae is found?

A. Older osteogenesis imperfecta case
B. More severe osteogenesis imperfecta
C. Both of the above
D. None of the above

7. **Caffey's disease is also known as:**
   A. Craniofacial dysostosis
   B. Mandibulofacial dysostosis
   C. Generalized cortical hyperostosis
   D. Infantile cortical hyperostosis

8. **Bone (s) most frequently affected in Caffey's disease is/ are:**
   A. Femur
   B. Mandible
   C. Clavicle
   D. Both (B) and (C)

9. **Marie and Sainton's disease is also known as:**
   A. Craniofacial dysostosis
   B. Cleidocranial dysplasia
   C. Mandibulofacial dysostosis
   D. Infantile cortical hyperostosis

10. **Numerous unerupted supernumerary teeth are found in:**
    A. Generalized cortical hyperostosis
    B. Treacher Collins syndrome
    C. Crouzen syndrome
    D. Mutational dysostosis

11. **Most common craniosynostotic syndrome occurring with syndactyly is:**
    A. Crouzen syndrome
    B. Apert syndrome
    C. Pierre Robin syndrome
    D. van Buchem's syndrome

12. **All of the following are features of Treacher Collins syndrome *except*:**
    A. Antimongoloid palpebral fissures with a coloboma of the outer portion of upper lids
    B. Hypoplasia of malar bones
    C. Blind fistulas between the angles of the ears and the angles of the mouth
    D. Facial clefts

13. At which stage of embryo failure does differentiation of maxillary mesoderm result in Treacher Collins syndrome?

A. Embryo length 32 mm B. Embryo length 25 mm
C. Embryo length 50 mm D. Embryo length 62 mm

14. Goldenhar syndrome is:

A. Gardner's syndrome B. Hemifacial microsomia
C. Franceschetti syndrome D. Marfan syndrome

15. Pierre Robin syndrome consists of all these abnormalities *except*:

A. Cleft lip B. Cleft palate
C. Micrognathia D. Glossoptosis

16. "Bird facies" appearance is found in:

A. Arachnodactyly B. Robin anomalad
C. Crouzen syndrome D. Mandibulofacial dysostosis

17. Abraham Lincoln suffered from:

A. Crouzen syndrome B. Marble bone disease
C. Marfan syndrome D. Parkinsonism

18. Collagen is abnormally soluble in:

A. Arachnodactyly
B. Achondroplasia
C. Mandibulofacial dysostosis
D. Osteogenesis imperfecta

19. Among the following mandible is more commonly affected by:

A. Paget's disease B. Franceschetti's syndrome
C. Craniofacial dysostosis D. Marfan syndrome

20. All of the following are features of Marfan syndrome *except*:

A. High arched palate
B. Multiple Supernumerary teeth
C. Multiple odontogenic cysts of the maxilla
D. Bifid uvula

21. Most common chromosomal abnormality to occur in man is:

A. Dentinogenesis imperfecta B. Klinefelter's syndrome
C. Down's syndrome D. Marfan syndrome

22. All of the following are features of Down's syndrome *except*:

A. Small slanting eyes with epicanthal folds
B. Increased incidence of chronic leukemia
C. Prognathism
D. Hypermobility of the joints

23. Osteopetrosis is also known as:

A. Brittle bone disease B. Marble bone disease
C. Both of the above D. Lobestein disease

24. Albers-Schönberg disease is also known as:

A. Osteoporosis
B. Osteomalacia
C. Osteogenesis imperfecta
D. Osteopetrosis

25. Daily dietary requirement of vit. D is:

A. 200 IU of vitamin D B. 100 IU of vitamin D
C. 400 IU of vitamin D D. 800 IU of vitamin D

26. Which of the following is/are feature(s) of Osteopetrosis?

A. Elevated serum acid phosphatase level
B. Endosteal production of bone with an apparent concomitant lack of physiologic bone resorption
C. Both of the above
D. Benign form of osteopetrosis is a recessively inherited form

27. Which type of jaw relation is found in achondroplasia?

A. Class I
B. Class II division 2
C. Class III
D. Class II division 1

28. Death in patient of marble bone disease is due to:

A. Anemia
B. Secondary infection
C. Both of the above
D. Pathological fracture

29. Cranial nerve involvement due to narrowing of the cranial foramina is found in:

A. Osteopetrosis and osteomyelitis
B. Benign and malignant forms of osteopetrosis
C. Osteopetrosis and osteoporosis
D. Osteoporosis and osteomyelitis

30. Which type of anemia is found in Albers-Schönberg disease?

A. Hemolytic anemia
B. Iron deficiency anemia
C. Pernicious anemia
D. Myelophthisic anemia

31. Most commonly dwarfism occur in:

A. Down's syndrome
B. Achondroplasia
C. Crouzen syndrome
D. Treacher Collins syndrome

32. Which of the following is/are feature(s) of achondroplasia?

A. Disturbances in epiphyseal cartilage of long bones
B. Retardation of the zone of provisional calcification of endochondral growth
C. Brachycephalic face
D. All of the above

33. Osteitis deformans is also known as:

A. Paget's disease of bone
B. Achondroplasia
C. Osteogenesis imperfecta
D. Generalized cortical hyperostosis

34. Most commonly involved bone in osteitis deformans is:

A. Skull
B. Pelvis
C. Sacrum
D. Spine

35. "Cotton-wool" appearance in radiograph of skull and jaws is found in:

A. Paget's disease of bone B. Achondroplasia
C. Osteitis deformans D. Both (A) and (C)

36. Radiographic change(s) found in teeth in Paget's disease of bone is/are:

A. Resorption of root
B. Hypercementosis
C. Both of the above
D. Widening of periodontal ligament space

37. Which of the following values is increased in osteitis deformans?

A. Serum phosporus level
B. Serum calcium level
C. Serum acid phosphatase
D. Serum alkaline phosphatase

38. Serum alkaline phosphatase level in osteoblastic phase in increased up to:

A. 50 Bodansky unit B. 200 Bodansky unit
C. 250 Bodansky unit D. 350 Bodansky unit

39. Histologically, formation of "mosaic" bone is characteristic feature of:

A. Fibrous dysplasia B. Osteitis deformans
C. Both of the above D. Cherubism

40. Most serious complication of osteitis deformans is:

A. Pathological fracture
B. Skeletal deformity
C. Auditory and visual disturbance
D. Osteosarcoma

41. Most commonly affected bone in various syndromes and vanishing bone is:

A. Mandible B. Clavicle
C. Scapula D. Sacrum

42. van Buchem's disease is also known as:

A. Generalized cortical hyperostosis
B. Infantile cortical hyperostosis
C. Fibrous dysplasia of bone
D. Cherubism

43. Which of the following diseases is/are related to an active hyperemia of bone?

A. Phantom bone
B. Vanishing bone
C. Disappearing bone
D. All of the above

44. Etiology of fibrous dysplasia of bone is:

A. Genetic
B. Unknown
C. Environmental
D. Trauma

45. Most common presenting skeletal symptom during onset of fibrous dysplasia is:

A. Swelling of bone
B. Aching recurrent bone pain
C. Spontaneous fracture of bone
C. None of the above

46. Vaginal bleeding at the age of two or three years is found in case of:

A. Cherubism
B. Monostotic fibrous dysplasia
C. Polystotic fibrous dysplasia
D. Paget's disease of bone

47. Radiographic appearance in polystotic fibrous dysplasia is:

A. Cotton wool appearance
B. Unilocular cystic appearance
C. Uncertain
D. Multilocular cystic appearance

48. Familial fibrous dysplasia of the jaws is known as:

A. Polystotic fibrous dysplasia
B. Monostotic fibrous dysplasia
C. Cherubism
D. Vanishing bone

49. All of the following features characterize familial fibrous dysplasia of the jaws *except*:

A. Progressive painless symmetrical swelling of the maxilla and mandible
B. Deciduous dentition shed as early as three years of age
C. In jaws teeth floating in cystlike spaces are present
D. Presence of large multinucleated giant cells

50. Which type of malocclusion occurs if Still's disease involves the temporomandibular joint?

A. Class II division 1 **B.** Class II division 2
C. Class III **D.** Class I division 1

51. Fibrous ankylosis of TMJ occurs in:

A. Trauma to temporomandibular joint (TMJ)
B. Arthritis of temporomandibular joint
C. Rheumatoid arthritis of TMJ
D. Osteoarthritis

52. Among the following muscles which is least affected in myofascial pain-dysfunction syndrome?

A. Lateral pterygoid
B. Masseter
C. Temporalis
D. Medial Pterygoid

53. Which of the following features is not related to myofascial pain-dysfunction syndrome?

A. Etiology is related to "psycho-physiologic theory"
B. Females are more commonly affected than males
C. Muscle tenderness is most common over angle of mandible
D. Treatment of this syndrome is conservative

Explanations

1.D. The chief clinical characteristic of osteogenesis imperfecta is the extreme fragility and porosity of the bones, with an attendant proneness to fracture.

2.D. The form of osteogenesis imperfecta present in childhood is known as tarda or Lobstein's type, gravis or levis.

3.C. Hyperplastic callus formation, which may or may not be related to actual fracture, occasionally occurs in some patients.

4.D. Blue sclera is also seen in osteopetrosis, Marfan syndrome as well as in normal infants.

5.C. The basic defect appears to lie in the organic matrix with failure of fetal collagen to be transformed into mature collagen; calcification proceeds normally.

6.C. White sclerae are generally found in the older patients with the more severe disease and earlier onset of fractures.

7.D. Caffey's disease is also known as Caffey-Silverman syndrome.

8.D. Other bones which commonly demonstrate hyperostosis are the calvarium, scapula, ribs and tubular bones of the extremeties, including the metatarsals.

9.B. It is also known as mutational dysostosis.

10.D. These are most prevalent in the mandibular premolar and incisor areas.

11.B. Most common of the craniosynostotic syndromes occurring without syndactyly is craniofacial dysostosis, or crouzon disease.

12.A. The characteristic facies of the patients have often been described as being bird like or fish like in nature. The coloboma is present on the outer portion of lower lid.

13.C. Treacher Collins syndrome is also known as mandibulo-facial dysostosis.

14.B. Also known as oculoauriculovertebral dysplasia.

15.A. Other systemic finsings may also be present in the Pierre Robin syndrome, including congenital heart defects, other skeletal anomalies and ocular lesions.

16.B. Robin anomalad is another name of Pierre Robin syndrome.

17.C. The outstansing characteristic of Marfan syndrome is the excessive length of the tubular bones or disproportionately long thin extremeties.

18.A. Arachnodactly is another name of Marfan syndrome.

19.B. Franceschetti syndrome is also known as mandibulofacial dysostosis.

20.B. Marfan syndrome is basically a disease of connective tissue related to a defective organization of collagen.

21.C. In Down's syndrome, there is trisomy of chromosome No 21.

22.B. It is of significant interest that individuals with down's syndrome, especially children, have an increased incidence of acute leukemia.

23.B. Osteopetrosis is also known as Albers-Schönberg disease.

24.D. Osteopetrosis is of two types–malignant recessive and benign dominant.

25.C.

26.C. The predominance of bone formation over resorption typically leads to the persistence of cartilaginous cores of bony trabeculae.

27.C. The maxilla is retruded because of restriction of growth of the base of the skull, and the retrusion may produce a relative mandibular prognathism.

28.C. No known patient with osteopetrosis has survired past the age of 20 years.

29.B. Cranial nerve involvement in both types of the disease is a result of narrowing of the cranial foramina by bone deposition with resultant impingement on the nerves.

30.D. The patients manifest a myelophthisic anemia due to the displacement of hemopoisetic marrow tissue by bone.

31.B. He is quite short, usually under 1.4 meters, with short and thickened muscular extremities, a brachy cephalic skull and bowed legs.

32.D. It is a hereditary condition that is transmitted as an autosomal dominant characteristic.

33.A. Bone in osteitis deformans is extremely vascular, and it has been suggested that the vessels are similar to arteriovenous aneurysms.

34.C. Most commonly involved bone in osteitis deformans is sacrum followed by spine and right femur.

35.D. The osteoblastic areas appears as opacities in the roentgenogram, tend to be patchy in distribution, eventually becoming confluent, but often still showing minute areas of variation in radiodensity. The patchiness has been termed as 'cotton wool appearance.'

36.C. The roentgenographic features of osteitis deformans are varied and depend upon the stage of the disease encountered.

37.D. Values as high as over 250 Bodansky units have been reported, particularly in patients in the ostcoblastic phase of the disease, when there is rapid formation of new bone and when there is polyostotic involvement.

38.C. In the monostotic form of the disease, the alkaline phosphatase level seldom exceeds 50 Bodansky units.

39.B. Mosaic bone is a descriptive term used to indicate the appearance of bone, which has been partially resorbed and then repaired, leaving deeply staining hematoxyphilic reversal lines.

40.D. Complications may arise related to the bony alterations, including pathologic fractures the skeletal deformities and the auditory and visual disturbances.

41.B. Most commonly affected bones in vanishing bone are the clavicle, scapula, humerus, ribs, ilium, ischium and sacrum.

42.A. Van buchem disease is also known as endosteal hyperostosis.

43.D. Massive ostealysis is an unusual and uncommon disease characterized by spontaneous, progressive resorption of bone with ultimate total disappearance of the bone.

44.B. Fibrous dysplasia of bone is one of the most perplexing diseases of osseous tissue. It is a lesion of unknown etiology, uncertain pathogenesis and diverse histopathology.

45.B. The disease usually manifests itself early in life with an evident deformity, bowing or thickening of long bones, often unilateral in distribution.

46.C. The female patients, but not males, exhibit precocious puberty, sometimes beginning at the age of two or three years or even younger .

47.D. In polyostotic fibrous dysplasia, the medullary portions of bone are rarefied and present irregular trabeculations, often a multilocular cystic appearance.

48.C. Cherubism is also known as familial fibrous swelling of the jaws.

49.A. Patient exhibits a progressive, painless, symmetric swelling of the jaw, mandible or maxilla, producing the typical chubby face suggestive of a cherub.

50.A. Rheumatoid arthnitis in children (Still's disease), when involves the temporomandibular joint, may cause a malocclusion of the class II division I type with protrusion of maxillary incisors and anterior open bite.

51.C. Occasionally the connective tissue becomes ossified and a true bony ankylosis occur.

52.D. The specific muscles affected are the lateral pterygoid (in 84%cases), masseter (in 70%), temporalis (in 49%), medial pterygoid (in 35%) and the cervical, scalp and facial.

53.C. There are 4 cardinal signs and symptoms of the syndrome: (i) pain (ii) muscle tenderness, (iii)clicking or popping noise in the TMJ, and (iv) limitation of jaw motion, unilaterally or bilaterally , sometimes with deviation on opening .

15

Diseases of the Blood and Blood Forming Organs

1. Biermer's anemia is also known as:

A. Primary anemia
B. Mediterranean disease
C. Aplastic anemia
D. Iron deficiency anemia

2. Which of the following anemias is characterized by triad of symptoms-generalized weakness, a sore painful tongue and numbness or tingling of the extremities?

A. Aplastic anemia
B. Iron deficiency anemia
C. Addison's anemia
D. Cooley's anemia

3. "Bald tongue of sandwith" is seen in:

A. Biermer's anemia
B. Pellagra
C. Aplastic anemia
D. Mediterranean disease

4. Hunter's glossitis is found in:

A. Pernicious anemia
B. Cooley's anemia
C. Idiopathic steatorrhea
D. Aplastic anemia

5. Gastric carcinoma is associated with:

A. Sprue
B. Thalassemia
C. Erythroblastosis fetalis
D. Primary anemia

6. Treatment of pernicious anemia consists of:

A. Vitamin B_{12}
B. Folic acid
C. Both of the above
D. None of the above

7. Fanconi's syndrome is associated with:

A. Thalassemia
B. Aplastic anemia
C. Polycythemia rubra vera
D. Leukopenia

8. Hemoglobin H disease is a:

A. Homozygous β-thalassemia
B. Heterozygous β- thalassemia
C. Homozygous α- thalassemia
D. Heterozygous α- thalassemia

9. Which of the following is/are generally without clinical manifestation?

A. Thalassemia trait of α-thalassemia
B. Thalassemia trait of α-thalassemia
C. Both of the above
D. Thalassemia major of α-thalassemia

10. Malocclusion usually associated with thalassemia is:

A. Class I
B. Class II division 1
C. Class III
D. Class II division 2

11. Nucleated red blood cells are a characteristic feature of:

A. Aplastic anemia
B. Thalassemia
C. Pernicious anemia
D. Iron deficiency anemia

12. "Safety-Pin" cells are characteristic finding in:

A. Erythroblastic anemia
B. Sickle cell anemia
C. Both of the above
D. Aplastic anemia

13. In intraoral periapical radiograph "salt and pepper" effect is found in:

A. Aplastic anemia
B. Sickle cell anemia
C. Cooley's anemia
D. Iron deficiency anemia

14. In the heterozygote form of sickle cell anemia, hemoglobin S is:

A. 10% of total hemoglobin
B. 20% of total hemoglobin
C. 30% of total hemoglobin
D. 40% of total hemoglobin

15. In sickle cell anemia, which of the followings occurs?

A. Substitution of valine for glutamine at the sixth position of the α-globin chain
B. Substitution of glutamine for valine at the sixth position of the α-globin chain
C. Substitution of valine for glutamine at the sixth position of the β-globin chain
D. Substitution of glutamine for valine at the sixth position of the β-globin chain

16. Which of the following murmurs occurs in sickle cell anemia?

A. Systolic murmur B. Early diastolic murmur
C. Continuous murmur D. Mid diastolic murmur

17. "Hair-on-end" pattern in skull radiograph is found in:

A. Thalassemia
B. Congenital hemolytic jaundice
C. Chronic iron deficiency anemia
D. All of the above

18. Deoxygenated sickle hemoglobin molecule undergoes:

A. Gelation B. Crystallization
C. Any of the above D. None of the above

19. Most of the Rh-positive patients have:

A. C antigen B. D antigen
C. E antigen D. D antigen

20. Most of the Rh-negative patient have:

A. d-e antigen B. e-e antigen
C. d-d antigen D. c-c antigen

21. Anti-D gamma globulin injection given in case of erythroblastosis fetalis binds to:

A. Maternal red cells (antibody site)
B. Fetal red cells (antibody site)
C. Maternal red cells (antigenic site)
D. Fetal red cells (antigen site)

22. Test used for erythroblastosis fetalis is:

A. Positive indirect coombs test on fetal blood
B. Positive direct coombs test on fetal blood
C. Positive direct coombs test on cord blood
D. Positive indirect coombs test on cord blood

23. "Rh hump" found in erythroblastosis fetalis is:

A. Square defect B. Rectangular defect
C. Ringlike defect D. Ovoid defect

24. Plummer-vinson syndrome is associated with:

A. Iron deficiency anemia B. Thalassemia
C. Aplastic anemia D. Pernicious anemia

25. Relative polycythemia occurs in:

A. Bone marrow anoxia B. Chronic vomiting
C. Heart disease D. Both (A) and (C)

26. Which of the following is/are erythropoietic stimulatory factor (s)?

A. Gum shellac B. Phosphorous
C. Some liver carcinoma D. All of the above

27. Osler's disease is also known as:

A. Rendu-Osler-Weber disease
B. Hereditary hemorrhagic telengiectasia
C. Both of the above
D. Polycythemia vera

28. Which of the followings is not correct about erythremia?

A. Absolute increase in red cells and in total blood volume
B. Splenomegaly is one of the most constant feature
C. Color index is more than one
D. Bleeding and clotting times are normal

29. Which of the followings is also known as Vaquez's disease?

A. Cooley's anemia B. Leukopenia
C. Leukocytosis D. Osler's disease

30. Which of the followings can cause leukopenia?

A. Typhoid fever
B. Brucellosis
C. Measles
D. All of the above

31. Most common cause of agranulocytosis is:

A. Infection
B. Drugs
C. Genetic
D. None of the above

32. Agranulocytosis generally occurs in:

A. Infants
B. Adults
C. Old age
D. None of the above

33. Cyclic neutropenia is also known as:

A. Periodic neutropenia
B. Cyclic agranulocytic angina
C. Periodic agranulocytosis
D. All of the above

34. Etiology of cyclic neutropenia is/are:

A. Environmental
B. Genetic
C. Idiopathic
D. Hormonal

35. Periadenitis mucosa necrotica recurrens is found in:

A. Pellagra
B. Agranulocytic angina
C. Agranulocytosis
D. Leukopenia

36. Giant abnormal granules found in peripheral circulating leukocyte in Chediak-Higashi syndrome are basically altered:

A. Peroxisome
B. Ribosome
C. Mitochondria
D. Lysosome

37. Glandular fever is caused by:

A. Cytomegalo virus
B. Epstein Barr virus
C. Herpes zoster
D. None of the above

38. Which of the following is/are caused by Epstein barr virus?

A. Burkitt's African jaw lymphoma
B. Nasopharyngeal carcinoma
C. Lymphoblastic leukemia
D. All of the above

39. Which of the following is usually the first to exhibit enlargement in infectious Mononucleosis?

A. Cervical lymph nodes
B. Axillary lymph nodes
C. Groin lymph nodes
D. None of the above

40. Increased heterophil antibody titer is found in:

A. Kissing disease
B. Glandular fever
C. Both of the disease
D. Darling's disease

41. Which of the following pharyngeal lesions is most common in case of infectious mononucleosis?

A. Sore throat
B. Pharyngitis
C. Tonsillitis
D. Enlarged tonsils and pharyngeal lymphoid tissue

42. Which of the followings is most common oral lesion in infectious mononucleosis?

A. Oral ulceration
B. Oral palatal petechiae
C. Acute stomatitis and gingivitis
D. Oral membrane, focal or extensive

43. Survival span in acute form of leukemia is:

A. Less than six months
B. Less than one year
C. Less than five years
D. Between six months and one year

44. Philadelphia chromosome is found in:

A. Acute myeloid leukemia
B. Acute lymphoid leukemia
C. Chronic myeloid leukemia
D. Chronic lymphoblastic leukemia

45. Which of the followings is correct about Philadelphia chromosome?

A. Translocation of chromosomal material from chromosome 21 to chromosome 9
B. Translocation of chromosomal material from chromosome 9 to chromosome 21
C. Translocation of chromosomal material from chromosome 22 to chromosome 9
D. Translocation of chromosomal material from chromosome 9 to chromosome 22

46. Which of the followings forms the basis for the final diagnosis of any type of leukemia?

A. Clinical examination
B. Hematological examination
C. Histopathological examination of lymph node
D. Radiographic findings

47. Which of the followings is/are characteristic of acute leukemia?

A. Anemia alone
B. Thrombocytopenia alone
C. Thromocytosis alone
D. Both (A) and (B)

48. Coagulation factor nine is:

A. Plasma thromboplastin antecedent (PTA)
B. Serum prothrombin conversion accelerator
C. Christmas factor
D. Labile factor

49. Aldrich syndrome is characterized by all of the followings *except*:

A. Poor antibody response to polysaccharide antigens
B. Normal antibody response to protein antigens
C. Serum IgM levels are high
D. Both qualitative and quantitative abnormality of the platelets

50. Hemophilia B occurs due to deficiency of:

A. Coagulation factor 8 B. Coagulation factor 9
C. Coagulation factor 11 D. Coagulation factor 5

51. Bleeding time is prolonged in:

A. von Willebrand's disease
B. Plasma thromboplastin antecedent deficiency
C. Hemophilia B
D. Deficiency of coagulation factor VII

52. Clotting time and prothrombin time are infinite in:

A. Dysfibrinogenemia B. Parahemophilia
C. Afibrinogenemia D. Macroglobulinemia

53. What is the value of erythrocyte sedimentation rate in case of afibrinogenemia?

A. One B. Infinite
C. Ten D. Zero

54. In which of the following diseases viscosity of the blood serum was usually extremely high?

A. Hypofibrinogenemia B. Macroglobulinemia
C. Dysfibrinogenemia D. Parahemophilia

55. Fibrin is stabilized by:

A. Gelation B. Crystallization
C. Both of the above D. Transamidation

56. Paradoxical thrombosis occurs in:

A. Dysfibrinogenemia B. Macroglobulinemia
C. Afibrinogenemia D. Parahemophilia

57. Parahemophilia occurs due to deficiency of:

A. Tissue thromboplastin B. Antihemophilic globulin
C. Proaccelerin D. Hageman factor

58. Which of the following patients suffering from leukemia do not manifest oral lesions?

A. Very old B. Very young children
C. Edentulous persons D. Both (B) and (C)

59. What is the value of heterophil titer in case of glandular fever?

A. 1:8 B. 1:4086
C. 1:4006 D. 1:4096

Explanations

1.A. Primary anemia is also known as pernicious anemia.

2.C. Other typical complaints are easy fatigability, headache, dizziness, nausea, vomiting, diarrhea, loss of appetite, shortness of breath, loss of weight, pallor and abdominal pain.

3.B. Advanced cases of pernicious anemia show smooth or bald tongue which is often referred to as Hunter's glossitis or Moeller's glossitis and is similar to the bald tongue of Sandwith seen in pellagra.

4.A. Hunter's glossitis is also known as Moeller's glossitis.

5.D. Achlorhydria, or lack of gastric hydrochloric acid secretion is a constant feature of the disease, and the pH of the gastric contents is usually high.

6.C. Persons suffering from pernicious anemia have gastric juice which dose not not contain the "intrinsic factor" and therefore, they are unable to absorb distary vitamin B_{12}.

7.B. Fanconi's syndrome consists of congenital, and sometimes familial, aplastic anemia associated with a variety of other congenital defects including bone abnormalities, microcephaly and hypogenitalism.

8.C. Hemoglobin H disease is a very mild form of the disease in which the patient may live a relatively normal life.

9.C. In heterozygotes, the disease is mild and is called thalassemia minor or thalassemia trait.

10.B. The face often develops mongoloid features due to prominence of the cheek bones, protrusion or flaring of the maxillary anterior teeth.

11.B. The presence of typical safety-pin cells and of cormoblasts or nucleated red blood cells in the circulating blood is a characteristic feature of thalassemia.

12.A. Erythroblastic anemia is also known as thalassemia.

13.C. Intraoral roentgenograms in some cases reveal a peculiar trabecular pattern of the maxilla and mandible, characterized by an apparent coarsening of some trabeculae and the blurring and disappearance of others, resulting in a salt and pepper effect.

14.D. In the herterozygote, only about 40% of the hemoglobin is HbS, so that the individual has only the sickle cell trait and manifests clinical evidence of sickling only under conditions of severe hypoxia.

15.C. Sickle cell anemia is a hereditary type of chronic hemolytic anemia transmitted as a mendelian dominant and non-sex linked characteristic.

16.A. Cardiomegaly also occurs.

17.D. Hair on end pattern is also seen in sickle cell anemia, and secondary polycythemia of cyanotic congenital heart disease.

18.C. The sickle hemoglobin molecule undergoes gelation or crystallization when it is deoxygenated, and this physically distorts the erythrocyte, producing the sickle shape.

19.B. The 85 percent of the population generally considered Rh-positive actually have the D antigen homozygously (D-D) or heterozygously (D-d).

20.C. The 15 percent who are Rh negative have the d antigen homozygously (d-d).

21.D. Rh negative mothers are being given anti-D gamma globilin to prevent immunization, since it binds to antigenic receptor sites on fetal red cells, making them nonimmunogenic.

22.C. Erythroblastosis fetalis may be manifested in the teeth by the deposition of blood pigment in the enamel and dentin of the developing teeth, giving them a green, brown or blue hue.

23.C. Enamel hypoplasia usually involves the incisal edges of the anterior teeth and the middle portion of deciduous cuspid and first moloar crown. Hence, a characteristic ring like defect occurs.

24.A. The plummer vinson syndrome is one manifestation of iron deficiency anemia and was first described by Plummer in 1914.

25.B. Retative polycythemia is an apparent increase in the number of circulating red blood cells that occurs as a result of loss of body fluid with hemoconcentration of cells.

26.D. Erythropoietic stimulating factors also include various metals such as manganese, mercury, iron bismuth, arsenic and cobalt.

27.D. Polychythemia vera is also known as Vaquez's disease.

28.C. The color index is less than 1.

29.D. No specific treatment for Osler's disease is known.

30.D. Other causes of leukopenia include debilitating states, hemopoietic disorders, physical and chemical agents etc.

31.B. Most common drugs which causes agranulocytosis are amidopyrine, barbiturates, DDT, quinine, sulfonamides etc.

32.B. Agranulocytosis occurs at any age, but is somewhat more common in adults, particularly women.

33.D. Cyclic neutropeuia is an unusual form of agranulocytosis characterized by a periodic or cyclic diminution in circulating polymorphonuclear neutrophilic leukocytes.

34.C. A chronic idiopathic neutropenia, non-cyclic and nonfamilial, associated with severe persistent gingivitis has been reported.

35.B. Periadenitis mucosa necrotica recurrens may actually be cyclic neutropenia.

36.D. These granules are the hallmark of the syndrome and are invariably present.

37.B. Epstein-Barr virus is a herpes like virus which is the same virus that has been implicated as the etiologic agent in Burkitt's African jaw lymphoma and nasopharyngcal carcinoma.

38.D. Infectious mononucleosis is also caused by Epstein-Barr virus.

39.A. The cervical lymph nodes are usually the first to exhibit enlargement, followed by the nodes of the axilla and groin.

40.C. The patient exhibits atypical lymphocytes in the circulating blood, as well as antibodies to the EB virus and an increased heterophil antibody titer.

41.A. Other lesions include pharyngitis and tonsillitis, enlarged tonsils and pharyngeal lymphoid tissue and faucial and pharyngeal membrane.

42.C. The oral manifestations consisted chiefly of acute gingivitis and stomatitis, the appearance of white or gray membrane in various areas, palatal petechiae and occasional oral ulcers.

43.A. Chronic leukemia implies a survival of over one year.

44.C. Philadelphia chromosome is a translocation of chromosomal material from chromosome 22 to chromosome 9.

45.C. This chromosome disappears from the circulation during remission of the disease in many cases but will reappear when there is a relapse.

46.B. It is recognized, however, that subleukemic or aleukemic forms of the disease exist in which the white blood cell count of peripheral blood is normal or even subnormal.

47.D. As a result both bleeding time and coagulation time are prolonged.

48.C. Christmas factor is also known as plasma thromboplastin component

49.C. Serum IgM levels are low, but IgA and IgE levels may be normal or elevated.

50.B. A deficiency of factor VIII results in the occurrence of hemophilia A, which is the most common type of hemophilia.

51.A. Bleeding times of over 300 minutes have been recorded, but more often they range between several minutes and one hour.

52.C. The peripheral blood fails to clot even after the addition of thrombin.

53.D. The cells remaining suspended even after 24 hours.

54.B. Frequent gelling of the serum upon cooling to room temperature or lower.

55.D. Activated factor XIII cross links fibrin or stabilizes it by transamidation.

56.A. The disease manifests itself clinically by a mild to severe bleeding tendency although, interestingly, paradoxical thrombosis has also been reported.

57.C. Proaccelerin is responsible for the conversion of prothrombin to thrombin.

58.D. Infrequency of oral manifestations in childhood leukemia is due primarily to the high incidence of acute hymphocytic leukemia in this age group, since this type is least likely to produce oral lesions.

59.D. The normal titer of agglutinins and hemolysins in human blood against sheep red blood cells does not exceed 1:8.

16

Diseases of the Periodontium

1. Which of the followings represent/s dystrophy?

A. Periodontitis
B. Gingivosis
C. Gingivitis
D. Both (B) and (C)

2. The color of the normal gingiva is:

A. Cool pink
B. Red
C. Coral pink
D. Light pink

3. Which of the followings cause (s) mesial drift?

A. Stresses of occlusion
B. Pressure of tongue
C. Pressure from facial musculature
D. All of the above

4. Largest group of periodontal fibers is:

A. Apical fibers
B. Oblique fibers
C. Horizontal fibers
D. Alveolar crest fiber

5. Maximum number of epithelial rests of malassez is/are found in:

A. Apical area in first and second decades of life
B. Cervical area throughout the life
C. Both of the above
D. Apical area throughout the life

6. The width of the periodontal ligament of teeth in function is:

A. 0.10 to 0.15 mm
B. 0.20 to 0.25 mm
C. 0.25 to 0.40 mm
D. 0.40 to 0.50 mm

7. Acquired pellicle reaches its mature thickness within:

A. 30 minutes
B. One hour
C. Ten hours
D. 24 hours

8. Thickness of mature acquired pellicle is:

A. 0.01 to 0.08 microns
B. 0.1 to 0.8 microns
C. 1.0 to 1.8 microns
D. 0.25 to 0.40 microns

9. Which of the following stains is dominated by *Actinomyces species*?

A. Brown stain
B. Green stain
C. Black stain
D. Orange stain

10. Which of the followings is not correct about calculus?

A. Subgingival calculus is also known as "serumal calculus"
B. Supragingival calculus in harder than subgingival calculus
C. Subgingival calculus is more brittle
D. Subgingival calculus is much denser

11. By which of the following mechanisms calculus is attached to the tooth?

A. Attachment to microscopic irregularities on the cementum
B. Attachment into areas of cementum resorption
C. Attachment to the secondary dental cuticle
D. All of the above

12. Which of the followings is/are feature (s) of acute necrotising ulcerative gingivitis?

A. Interdental papilla is covered by grey, necrotic pseudomembrane
B. Typical fetid odour
C. Metallic taste
D. All of the above

13. Which of the following microorganisms causes (s) trench mouth?

A. Fusiform bacilli
B. *Borrelia vincentii*
C. Both of the above
D. None of the above

14. Which of the followings is/are an ideal location for reinfection of vincent's infection?

A. Incubation zone
B. Flap of erupting third molar
C. Both of the above
D. None of the above

15. All of the following features about Borrelia vincentii are true *except*:

A. Gram-negative spirochete
B. Nonmotile
C. Can be cultured anaerobically
D. Have three to six long loose spirals

16. The final diagnosis of trench mouth is dependent on:

A. Histopathological examination
B. Radiographic evaluation
C. Bacteriological examination
D. Clinical examination

17. Inflammatory hyperplasia can be associated with:

A. Vitamin C deficiency
B. Endocrine imbalance
C. Crohn's disease
D. All of the above

18. Most favorable type of pocket for reattachment is:

A. One wall infrabony pocket
B. Two wall infrabony pocket
C. Three wall infrabony pocket
D. Suprabony pocket

19. A "slanting fill-in" of bone can occur in a:

A. Three wall infrabony pocket
B. Two wall infrabony pocket
C. One wall infrabony pocket
D. Suprabony pocket

20. Earliest change in the periodontal bone in periodontitis is:

A. Resorption of buccal or labial bone
B. Resorption of lingual bone
C. Blunting of the alveolar crest
D. Formation of intrabony pocket

21. Parulis is also known as:

A. Gum boil

B. Apical periodontal abscess

C. Lateral periodontal abscess

D. Both (A) and (C)

22. Which of the followings is/are desquamative gingivitis?

A. Lichen planus B. Pemphigus

C. Cicatricial pemphigoid D. All of the above

Explanations

1.B. Periodontal diseases are classified into two general groups on the basis of the pathologic processes present: (i) inflammation (gingivitis and periodontitis), and (ii) dystrophy (gingivosis and periodontosis).

2.C. The color of the normal gingiva is a pale, coral pink, and in the adult the tissue is dense,firm to the touch and insensitive to moderate pressure.

3.D. During adulthood, the teeth are constantly subjected to the stresses of occlusion as well as to those of the tongue and facial musculature which may prompt that tooth movement called mesial drift.

4.B. Oblique fibers which extend from the cementum coronally toward the alveolar bone and constitute the largest group.

5.C. Greater persistence of epithelial rests in the cervical area may be correlate with and influenced by the constant inflammatory reaction present in the area of gingival sulcus.

6.C. The width of the periodontal ligament of teeth in function (0.25 to 0.40) is much greater than the very thin periodontal ligament (0.10 to 0.15 mm).

7.D. The acquired pellicle is a thin deposit which may form shortly after eruption on the exposed surfaces of teeth.

8.B. Acquired pellicle is free of bacteria and completely covers the tooth surface.

9.C. The deposit is easily removed and often recurs slowly.

10.B. Supragingival calculus is also known as salivary calculus.

11.D. Attachment also occurs by penetration of microorganisms of the calculus matrix into the cementum.

12.D. Acute necrotizing ulcerative gingivitis is also known as trench mouth.

13.C. Acute necrotizing ulcerative gingivitis is a primany disease caused by a fusiform bacillus and *Borrelia vincentii*, a spirochete, coexisting in a symbiotic relationship.

14.C. After healing of acute necrotizing ulcerative gingivitis, the crests of the interdental papillae which have been destroyed, leaving a hollowed out area, constitute an area which retains debris and microorganisms, and can serve as an "incubation zone."

15.B. *Borrelia vincentii* measures approximately 10 to 15 microns in length.

16.D. Athough the bacterial smear may be of value as an aid in diagnosis of atypical cases of acute necrotizing ulcerative gingivitis, the final diagnosis is a clinical one.

17.D. Inflammatory hyperplasia of the gingiva usually results from chronic inflammation of the gingival tissues.

18.C. Reattachment may be defined as a re-establishment of fibrous connection of tooth to alveolar bone and gingiva by periodontal fibers in an area of cementum, which was adjacent to a pathologic pocket.

19.B. But when only one wall is present, chances for formation of additional height of alveolar bone are poor.

20.C. As resorption progresses, there is horizontal loss of more bone, often with a tendency for a cupping out of the interdental alveolar bone.

21.D. A direct incision perpendicular to the long axis of the involved tooth will release pus, while the introduction of a periodontal pocket probe from the gingiva to the area will release the pus around the neck of the tooth.

22.D. Cicatrical pemphigoid is also known as benign mucous membrane pemphigoid.

17

Diseases of the Skin

1. Which of the followings is/are found in hereditary ectodermal dysplasia?

A. Hypohydrosis
B. Hypotrichosis
C. Hypodontia
D. All of the above

2. Hereditary ectodermal dysplasia is:

A. Autosomal dominant disease
B. Autosomal recessive disease
C. X-linked recessive disease
D. X-linked dominant disease

3. In which of the following diseases first symptom is development of unexplained fever with elevation of temperature?

A. Ellis-van Creveld syndrome
B. Lichen planus
C. Hereditary ectodermal dysplasia
D. Keratosis follicularis

4. Which of the followings is not a feature of hereditary ectodermal dysplasia?

A. Sebaceous gland is normal but mustache are usually abnormal
B. Bridge of the nose is depressed
C. Patients can be mistaken for siblings
D. Cone shaped teeth

5. All of the followings are correct about hereditary ectodermal dysplasia *except*:

A. The growth of jaws is impaired
B. Protuberant lips
C. Chronic refractory anemia
D. Deformed deciduous and permanent dentition

6. **In which of the following areas congenital absence of teeth is common in Ellis-van Creveld syndrome?**
   A. Maxillary anterior area
   B. Mandibular anterior area
   C. Maxillary posterior area
   D. Mandibular posterior area

7. **Wickham's striae are characteristic feature of:**
   A. Leukoplakia
   B. Erythroplakia
   C. Candidiasis
   D. Lichen planus

8. **Skin lesions of lichen planus occur on the:**
   A. Extensor surface
   B. Flexor surface
   C. Both of the above
   D. None of the above

9. **Which of the followings is not a feature of Grinspan's syndrome?**
   A. Hypertension
   B. Hypotension
   C. Diabetes mellitus
   D. Lichen planus

10. **Civatte bodies are found in:**
    A. Lichen planus
    B. Hereditary ectodermal dysplasia
    C. Dentigerous cyst
    D. Follicular cyst

11. **"Saw tooth" appearance of rete pegs is found in:**
    A. Dilantin hyerplasia
    B. Lichen planus
    C. Gingivitis
    D. Leukoplakia

12. **Civatte bodies are found in:**
    A. Spinous cell layer
    B. Basal cell layer
    C. Corneum stratum
    D. Both (A) and (B)

13. **Civatte bodies are:**
    A. Degenerated epithelial cells
    B. Phagocytosed epithelial cell remnants within microphages
    C. Both of the above
    D. Phagocytosed epithelial cell remnants within macrophages

14. Patchy linear pattern in direct immunofluorescence is found in

A. Lichen planus B. Lupus erythematosus
C. Erythema multiforme D. Pemphigus

15. Granular pattern in direct immunofluorescence is found in:

A. Pemphigus B. Pemphigoid
C. Lupus erythematosus D. Erythema multiforme

16. Which of the following oral lesions superficially resembles lichen planus?

A. Pemphigus B. Cicatricial pemphigoid
C. Lupus erythematosus D. All of the above

17. Epidermoid carcinoma is most common in:

A. Atrophic lichen planus B. Erosive lichen planus
C. Vesicular lichen planus D. Bullous lichen planus

18. Intralesional administration of corticosteroids is particularly important for:

A. Erosive lichen planus B. Bullous lichen planus
C. Vesicular lichen planus D. Atrophic lichen planus

19. Auspitz's sign is a feature of:

A. Pemphigus B. Psoriasis
C. Lichen planus D. Candidiasis

20. Psoriatic lesions are frequently found over skin on:

A. Flexor surface B. Extensor surface
C. Both of the above D. None of the above

21. The etiology of psoriasis is:

A. Genetic B. Environmental
C. Unknown D. Infection

22. Which of the followings is/are correct about psoriasis?

A. More severe in the winter
B. Less severe in the summer
C. Arthritis is a complication of psoriasis in some cases
D. All of the above

23. Which of the followings is not included in "psoriasiform" lesions?

- **A.** Ectopic geographic tongue
- **B.** Benign migratory glossitis
- **C.** Reiter's syndrome
- **D.** None of the above

24. Which of the following layers is absent in psoriasiform lesion?

- **A.** Stratum granulosum
- **B.** Stratum spinosum
- **C.** Stratum basale
- **D.** Stratum corneum

25. Normal skin turnover time is approximately:

- **A.** 21 days
- **B.** 24 days
- **C.** 28 days
- **D.** 34 days

26. 'Herald spot' is present in:

- **A.** Erythema multiforme
- **B.** Pityriasis rosea
- **C.** Kawasaki disease
- **D.** Keratosis follicularis

27. Turnover rate of epithelial cells in psoriatic skin is:

- **A.** 21 days
- **B.** 3 to 4 days
- **C.** 8 to 10 days
- **D.** 12 to 14 days

28. Which of the followings is correct about 'herald spot'?

- **A.** They are ovoid in shape
- **B.** Their long axis is perpendicular to the natural lines of cleavage of the skin
- **C.** They are secondary lesions
- **D.** All of the above

29. Most common precipitating agent for erythema multiforme is:

- **A.** Infectious mononucleosis
- **B.** Bacterial infection
- **C.** Barbiturate intake
- **D.** Herpes simplex infection

30. "Iris" lesions are found in:

A. Kawasaki disease
B. Keratosis follicularis
C. Stevens Johnson syndrome
D. Pityriasis rosea

31. Oral manifestations of which of the following diseases can be mistaken for acute necrotizing ulcerative gingivostomatitis?

A. Keratosis follicularis
B. Lichen planus
C. Candidiasis
D. Stevens-Johnson syndrome

32. Vesicles found in Stevens-Johnson syndrome are:

A. Intraepithelial
B. Subepithelial
C. Intradermal
D. All of the above

33. Lyell's disease is:

A. Pachyonychia congenita
B. Staphylococcal scalded skin syndrome
C. Toxic epidermal necrolysis
D. Darier's disease

34. Cardiac abnormality is the common complication of:

A. Erythema multiforme
B. Isolated Darier's disease
C. Mucocutaneous lymph node syndrome
D. Keratosis follicularis

35. Which of the following vitamins is associated with keratosis follicularis?

A. Vitamin B
B. Vitamin A
C. Vitamin D
D. Vitamin C

36. Corps ronds and grains are found in:

A. Pachyonychia congenita
B. Darier–White disease
C. Kawasaki disease
D. Isolated Darier's disease

37. In which of the following layers corps ronds are present?

A. Granular layer
B. Deep spinous cell layer
C. Both of the above
D. Stratum corneum layer

38. Grains are found in:

A. Spinous layer
B. Granular cell layer
C. Keratin layer
D. Basale layer

39. Corps ronds and grains are:

A. Fully keratinised cells
B. Partially keratinised cells
C. Basal cells
D. Giant cells present in granular cell layer

40. Typical suprabasilar cleavages are found in:

A. Darier-White disease
B. Warty dyskeratoma
C. Incontinentia pigmenti
D. Dyskeratosis congenita

41. What is the effect on turnover time of the epithelium in case of keratosis follicularis?

A. Decreased by twenty one fold
B. Decreased by seven fold
C. Increased by twenty one fold
D. Increased by seven fold

42. Warty dyskeratoma is also known as:

A. Isolated dyskeratosis follicularis
B. Isolated Darier's Disease
C. Both of the above
D. Bloch-Sulzberger syndrome

43. 'Cornoid lamella" is characteristic feature of:

A. Incontinentia pigmenti
B. Porokeratosis of Mibelli
C. Dyskeratosis congenita
D. Cannon's disease

44. Which of the followings is not a typical sign of dyskeratosis congenita?

A. Oral leukoplakia
B. Dystrophy of nails
C. Pigmentation of skin
D. Oral cancer

45. Which of the followings is associated with high incidence of cancer?

A. White sponge nevus
B. Porokeratosis of Mibelli
C. Dyskeratosis congenita
D. Incontinentia pigmenti

46. Which of the followings is most affected in acanthosis nigricans in oral cavity?

A. Buccal mucosa
B. Floor of mouth
C. Palate
D. Tongue

47. Nikolsky's sign is present in:

A. Pemphigus
B. Psoriasis
C. Erythema multiforme
D. Dyskeratosis congenita

48. Initial lesion of pemphigus foliaceus is:

A. Macule
B. Papule or pustule
C. Papillary projection
D. Bullous

49. Brazilian pemphigus is a mild endemic form of:

A. Pemphigus vegetans
B. Pemphigus foliaceus
C. Pemphigus erythematosus
D. Pemphigus vulgaris

50. Which of the following types has close resemblance to condyloma?

A. Pemphigus vegetans
B. Pemphigus foliaceus
C. Pemphigus erythematosus
D. Pemphigus vulgaris

51. All of the followings are wrong about pemphigus *except*:

A. Presence of intraepithelial vesicles
B. Presence of subepithelial vesicles
C. Presence of subbasilar split
D. Both (A) and (B)

52. "Dilapidated brick wall" effect is found in:

A. Benign mucous membrane pemphigoid
B. Familial benign chronic pemphigus
C. Bullous pemphigoid
D. Both (B) and (C)

53. Subepidermal vesicles are found in:

A. Parapemphigus B. Cicatricial pemphigoid
C. Both of the above D. Pemphigus vulgaris

54. Which of the following diseases show (s) a sensitivity to halogens?

A. Acrodermatitis enteropathica
B. Dermatitis herpetiformis
C. Both of the above
D. Lupus erythematosus

55. Which of the following cells differentiate dermatitis herpetiformis from erythema multiforme due to their more than ten percent presence?

A. Lymphocytes B. Basophils
C. Eosinophils D. Neutrophils

56. Butterfly distribution of patch on the malar regions and across the bridge of nose is found in:

A. Scalded skin syndrome
B. Discoid form of Lupus erythematosus
C. Pemphigus vulgaris
D. Erythema multiforme

57. Lupus erythematous cells are found in:

A. Systemic sclerosis
B. Ehlers–Danlos syndrome
C. Solar elastosis
D. Systemic lupus erythematosus

58. Masklike appearance of face is found in:

A. Scleroderma B. Solar elastosis
C. Hidebound disease D. Both (A) and (C)

59. Patient with which of the following disease/s is also known as 'Rubber man'?

A. Solar elastosis
B. Cutis hyperelastica
C. Actinic elastosis
D. Both (B) and (C)

60. Sailor's skin is found in:

A. Actinic keratosis
B. Senile elastosis
C. Both of the above
D. Goltz-Gorlin syndrome

61. Deficiency of lysyl hydroxylase is found in:

A. Ehlers-Danlos syndrome I
B. Ehlers-Danlos syndrome II
C. Ehlers-Danlos syndrome III
D. Ehlers-Danlos syndrome VI

62. Which type of collagen is defective in Ehlers-Danlos syndrome type IV?

A. Type I collagen
B. Type II collagen
C. Type III collagen
D. Type IV collagen

Explanations

1.D. Hereditary ectodermal dysplasia is a specific syndrome characterized by a congential dysplasia of one or more ectodermal structures and their accessory appendages manifested primarily by hypohidrosis, hypotrichosis and hypodontia.

2.C. Males being affected much more frequently than females.

3.C. Such persons cannot perspire, and they consequentty suffer from hyperpyrexia and an inability to tolerate warm temperatures.

4.A. The sebaceous glands and hair follicles are often defective or absent.

5.A. Dentures may be used even in relatively young patients, but they must be reconstructed periodically as the jaws contiune to grow.

6.B. Ellis-van Ceveld syndrome is also known as chondro-ectodermal dysplasia.

7.D. Wickham's striae are very fine grayish white lines.

8.B. Skin lesions occur most often on the flexor surfaces of the wrist and forearms, the inner aspect of the knees and thighs, and trunk, especially the sacral area.

9.B. An interesting association of lichen planus, diabetes melintis and vascular hypertension has been described by Grinspan, the triad being described as Grinspan's syndrome by Grupper.

10.A. Civatte bodies are present in the epithelium, mostly in the spinous and basal cell layers, appearing as sound, eosinophilic globules probably representing degenerated epithelial cells or phagocytosed epithelial cell remnants within microphages.

11.B. Other fingings include hyperparakeratosis or hyperorthokeratosis with thickening of the granular layer, acanthosis with intracellular edama of the spinous cells in some instances.

12.D. Civatte bodies are also known as colloid bodies or hyaline bodies also appear to correspond to structures called cytoid bodies.

13.C. Civatte bodies also appear to correspond to structures called cytoid bodies.

14.C. Patchy linear pattern in direct immunofluorescence is also found in pemphigoid.

15.A.

16.D. Other oral lesions, which bear superficial resemblance to lichen planus, include leukoplakia, condidiasis, erythema multiformal, and syphilis and recurrent aphthae.

17.B. An analogous malignant transformation of dermal lichen planus has been reported but is very rare.

18.A. Corticosteroid therapy has been used in severe cases to relieve the inflammation and decrease the prunitis of skin lesions.

19.B. If the deep scales are removed, one or more tiny bleeding points are disclosed, a characteristic feature termed Auspitz's sign.

20.B. Particularly the elbows and knees, the scalp, back and chest, face and abdomen.

21.C. Infection by various microorganisms, metabolic disturbance, endocrine dysfunction, neurogenic factors and trauma, as well as parturition, have been considered important precipitating factors.

22.D. Patients who move to a warm sunny climate usually undergo improvement in their condition.

Psoriatic involvement of oral mucosa is extremely rare and many oral lesions occurring concomitant with psoriasis of the skin are actually other diseaes such as leukoplakia or lichen planus.

24.A. The microscopic appearance of psoriasis is characterized by uniform parakeratosis, absence of stratum granulosum and elongation and clubbing of the rete pegs.

25.C. Normal skin turnover time is approximately 28 days while that of psoriatic skin is only 3 to 4 days.

26.B. Herald spot is brighter red and larger (3 to 4 cm in diameter) than the mutiple eruptions which follow its appearance.

27.B. The most commonly used topical medications are corticosteroids, tars and such drugs as iodochlor-hydroxyquin, dihydroxyanthralin and retinoic acid.

28.A. Herald spot is commonly ovoid, with the long axis parallel to the natural lines of cleavage of the skin, and are covered by a thin silvery scale.

29.D. The most common precipitating agent is herpes simplex infection preceding the onset of erythoma multiforme by one to three weeks.

30.C. A concentric ringlike appearance of the lesions, resulting from the varying shades of erythema are known as target, iris or bull's eye. They are most common on the hands, wrists and ankles.

31.D. In Stevens-Johnson syndrome mucosal vesieles or bullae occur which rupture and leave surfaces covered with a thick white or yellow exudates.

32.B. Cutaneous or mucosal lesions generally exhibit intracellular edema of the spinous layer of epithelium and edema of the superficial connective tissue, which may actually produced a subepidermal vesicle.

33.C. Toxic epidermal necrolysis is a very serious, often fatal, bullous drug eruption, so severe that large sheets of skin peel off, giving the appearance of a widespread scalding burn.

34.C. while the vast majority of cases are self-limiting and nonfatal, occasional deaths do occur almost invariably as a result of the cardiac complications, usually a coronary thrombosis or vascular damage related to infantile periarteritis nodosa.

35.B. Keratosis follicutaris has some relationship to vitamin A metabolism, since some patients have low plasma levels of the vitamin.

36.B. The corps rounds are larger than normal squamous cells and have a round, homogeneous, basophilic nucleus with dark eosinophilic cytoplasm and a distinct cell membrane.

37.A. Cops ronds are found usually in the granular layer and superficial spinous layer.

38.C. Grains are small, elongated parakeratotic cells situated in the keratin layer.

39.B. Both corps rounds and grains represent partially keratinized cells and are found also in the typical slit like intradermal vesicles just above the basal layer of cells, the typical suprabasilar cleavage.

40.A. Acantholytic cells are commonly found floating in the lacunae produced by this intraepithelial seperation.

41.B. The basic defect in epidermal synthesis, turnover and resultant keratinization is related to a defect in the desmosome-tonofilament complex.

42.C. The warty dyskeratoma is a lesion which bears marked histologic similarity to keratosis folliculoris, but, in contrast to the latter, is usually a single isolated focus.

43.B. The elevated horny margin of the lesion exhibits hyperkeratosis and acanthosis with a deep groove filled with parakeratin and a characteristic absence of the usual underlying granular layer.

44.D. Dyskeratosis congenital is a well recognized but rare genokeratosis which is probably inherited as a recessive characteristic with nearly all reported cares occurring in males.

45.C. High incidence of oral cancer develops in the young affected males.

46.D. There is hypertrophy of the filiform papillae producing a shaggy, papillomatous surface to the dorsal tongue.

47.A. The loss of epithelium occasioned by rubbing apparaently unaffected skin is termed Nikolsky's sign.

48.D. Pemphigus foliaceus is manifested by characteristic early bullous lesions which rapidly rupture and dry to leave masses of flakes or scales suggestive of an exfoliative dermatitis or eczema.

49.B. It often occurs in children and frequently in family groups. The course of the disease is similar to that of pemphigus foliaceus.

50.A. *Pemphigus vegetans* occur first on the nose and in the mouth, axillae and anogenital region and here bear close resemblance to condylomas.

51.A. Pemphigus as an entity is characterized microscopyically by the formation of a vesicle or bulla entirely intraepithelially, just above the basal layer producing the distinctive suprabasilar split.

52.B. Intercellular bridges persist so that adjacent epithelial cells still adhere to each other and are not entirely acantholylic. This appearance has been given the classic description of the dilapidated brick wall effect.

53.C. Parapemphiqus is also known as bullous pemphigoid.

54.B. Dermatitis herpetiformis show a sensitivity to the halogens (chlorine, bromine, iodine and fluorine) both by patch test and after ingestion.

55.C. Dermatitis herpetiformis is a rare, benign, chronic, recurrent dermatologic disease of unknown etiology.

56.B. The typical cutaneous lesions are slightly elevated red or purple macules that are often covered by gray or yellow adherent scales.

57.D. This cell, or yellow adherent scales.

58.D. Scleroderma also shows clawlike appearance to the hands.

59.B. The characteristic clinical features of this disease are the hyperelasticity of skin, hyperextensibility of the joints and fragilily of the skin and blood vessels resulting in exvessive bruising as well as defective healing of skin wounds.

60.B. Sailor's skin is also known as farmer's skin.

61.D. EDS VI is an autosomal recessive and characterized by a lysy 1 hydroxylase deficiency, so that the hydroxylysine content of skin is practically nil.

62.C. EDS IV is a clinically and genetically heterogeneous group in which there is an abnormality of type III collagen.

18

Diseases of Nerves and Muscles

1. What is the ratio of right and left side of face being affected in trigeminal neuralgia?

A. 1:5
B. 5:1
C. 1.7:1
D. 1.5:1

2. Which of the following nerves is mainly involved in Trotter's syndrome?

A. Ophthalmic nerve
B. Maxillary nerve
C. Mandibular nerve
D. Trochlear nerve

3. Which of the following divisions of 5th cranial nerve is mainly involved in postherpetic neuralgia?

A. Ophthalmic
B. Maxillary
C. Mandibular
D. Both (B) and (C)

4. Paratrigeminal syndrome is differentiated from Horner's syndrome by:

A. Presence of pain
B. Little or no change in sweating activity
C. Both of the above
D. None of the above

5. "Alarm clock" headache is seen in:

A. Vidian nerve neuralgia
B. Periodic migrainous neuralgia
C. Both of the above
D. Horner syndrome

6. Which of the following arteries is involved in Horton's syndrome?

A. External maxillary artery
B. Internal carotid artery
C. Internal maxillary artery
D. Inferior alveolar artery

7. Which of the followings is not a sphenopalatine neuralgia?

A. Sluder's headache
B. Meniere's disease
C. Meniere's syndrome
D. Periodic migrainous neuralgia

8. Orolingual paresthesia is caused by:

A. Pernicious anemia
B. Pellagra
C. Mercurialism
D. All of the above

9. Which of the followings is related to damage of auriculotemporal nerve?

A. Frey's syndrome
B. Gustatory sweating
C. Auriculotemporal syndrome
D. All of the above

10. "Crocodile tears" is associated with:

A. Frey's syndrome
B. Bell's palsy
C. Vidian nerve neuralgia
D. All of the above

11. Masklike face is associated with:

A. Seventh nerve paralysis
B. Sclerodrma
C. Both of the above
D. Trigeminal neuralgia

12. Bell's palsy is associated with:

A. Treacher Collins syndrome
B. Melkersson-Rosenthal syndrome
C. Cowden's syndrome
D. Raeder's syndrome

13. "Trigger zone" is found in:

A. Trigeminal neuralgia
B. Glossopharyngeal neuralgia
C. Multiple sclerosis
D. Both (A) and (B)

14. "Trigger zone" in glossopharyngeal neuralgia is situated in:

A. Posterior oropharynx B. Ala of the nose
C. Tonsillar fossa D. Both (A) and (C)

15. Staccato type of speech is found in:

A. Orofacial dyskinesia B. Glossopharyngeal neuralgia
C. Multiple sclerosis D. Migraine syndrome

16. Charcot's triad consists of all the following *except*:

A. Bladder incontinence B. Nystagmus
C. Dysarthria D. Intention tremor

17. Charcot's triad is a characteristic finding of:

A. Motor system disease B. Disseminated sclerosis
C. Both of the above D. Orofacial dyskinesia

18. Which of the followings is correct about multiple sclerosis?

A. Demyelinating disease affecting chiefly white matter of the peripheral nervous system
B. Demyelinating disease affecting mainly grey matter of the central nervous system
C. Demyelinating disease affecting mainly white matter of the central nervous system.
D. Demyelinating disease affecting mainly grey matter of the peripheral nervous system

19. Meniere's disease is characterized by:

A. Deafness B. Blindness
C. Stiffness of joint D. All of the above

20. In true Meniere's disease, there is:

A. Constriction of endolymphatic space and presence of inflammation
B. Constriction of endolymphatic space and absence of inflammation
C. Dilatation of endolymphatic space and presence of inflammation
D. Dilatation of endolymphatic space and absence of inflammation

21. Which of the followings is wrong about migraine?

A. Pain is usually bilateral
B. Pain is vascular in origin
C. Pain can occur in other side of head in successive attacks
D. Secondary effects are hormonal as well as neurogenic in origin

22. Ossification of the stylohyoid ligament causes:

A. Horner's disease
B. Jaw-winking syndrome
C. Eagle's syndrome
D. Marin Amat's syndrome

23. In Eagle's syndrome pain occurs along the distribution of:

A. Internal maxillary artery
B. Internal carotid artery
C. External carotid artery
D. Both (B) and (C)

24. Most consistent symptom of Eagle's syndrome is:

A. Laryngeal pain B. Pain in mandible
C. Pain in ear D. Pharyngeal pain

25. Which of the followings is absent in Horner's syndrome:

A. Mydriasis B. Ptosis
C. Anhidrosis D. Both (A) and (C)

26. Marcus Gunn phenomenon is also known as:

A. Marin Amat's syndrome B. Jaw-winking syndrome
C. Both of the above D. Eagle's syndrome

27. Which of the followings is not a primary myopathy?

A. Dystrophy B. Myotonia
C. Hypertrophy D. Both (B) and (C)

28. Which of the followings is a secondary myopathy?

A. Myositis B. Myasthenias
C. Atrophy D. Metabolic defects

29. Which of the followings is most common form of muscular dystrophy?

A. Severe generalized familial muscular dystrophy
B. Mild restricted muscular dystrophy
C. Myotonic dystrophy
D. Late distal muscular dystrophy

30. First affected muscles in severe generalized familial muscular dystrophy are:

A. Muscles of face
B. Muscles of extremities
C. Belly muscles
D. Muscles of neck

31. Enzyme increased in severe generalized familial muscular dystrophy is:

A. Serum alkaline phosphatase
B. Serum acid phosphatase
C. Serum phosphofructokinase
D. Serum creatine phosphokinase

32. "Tapir lips" is found in:

A. Mild restricted muscular dystrophy
B. Dystrophic myotonia
C. Acquired myotonia
D. Congenital myotonia

33. Mild restricted muscular dystrophy primarily involves:

A. Muscles of extremities
B. Muscles of face
C. Muscles of shoulders
D. Both (B) and (C)

34. "Myopathic facies" are found in:

A. Myotonic dystrophy
B. Late distal muscular dystrophy
C. Acquired myotonia
D. Congenital myotonia

35. Thomsen's disease is also known as:

A. Acquired myotonia
B. Congenital myotonia
C. Congenital dystrophy
D. Hemifacial spasm

36. Characteristic feature of congenital myotonia is myotonia associated with:

A. Muscular hyperplasia B. Muscular hypoplasia
C. Muscular hypertrophy D. Muscular hypotrophy

37. Herculean appearance is found in:

A. Myotonia congenita B. Paramyotonia
C. Myasthenia D. Muscular dystrophy

38. Cramping attack in case of paramyotonia is precipitated by:

A. Exposure to hot B. Exposure to cold
C. Percussion D. None of the above

39. "Floppy infant syndrome" is associated with:

A. Paramyotonia B. Hypotonia
C. Hemifacial spasm D. Dermatomyositis

40. Myasthenia gravis does not effect:

A. Skeletal muscle B. Smooth muscle
C. Cardiac muscle D. Both (B) and (C)

41. Sorrowful appearance of face is found in:

A. Progressive myositis ossificans
B. Bell's palsy
C. Myasthenia gravis
D. Hypotonia

42. "Swan neck" appearance is found in:

A. Dermatomyositis
B. Generalized myositis ossificans
C. Dystrophic myotonia
D. Acquired myotonia

43. Levels of which of the following enzyme (s) is/are increased in dermatomyositis?

A. Serum transaminase
B. Serum aldolase
C. Serum glucose-6-phosphase
D. Both (A) and (B)

44. "Petrified man" is found in:

A. Myositis ossificans circumscripta
B. Proliferative myositis
C. Focal myositis
D. Progressive myositis ossificans

45. Rider's bone is an example of:

A. Focal myositis
B. Ossifying hematoma
C. Traumatic ossifying myositis
D. Both (B) and (C)

46. Mobius syndrome is:

A. Congenital facial diplegia
B. Acquired Bell's palsy
C. Hemifacial microsomia
D. Hypertrophy of jaw muscles

47. Which of the following ocular muscles is mainly involved in Mobius syndrome?

A. Superior oblique B. Inferior oblique
C. Superior rectus D. Lateral rectus

48. Atrophy of muscles occurs in:

A. Denervation B. Vascular changes
C. Cachexia D. All of the above

49. Increase in size of muscle due to an increase in interstitial connective tissue, is known as:

A. Pseudohyperplasia of muscle
B. Pseudohypertrophy of muscle
C. Hypertrophy of muscle
D. Hyperplasia of muscle

50. Death in myasthenia gravis occurs due to:

A. Cardiac failure
B. Depression of central nervous system
C. Respiratory failure
D. All of the above

Explanations

1.C. It is a well established fact, but a completely unexplained one that the ringt side of the face is affected in more patients than the left by a ratio of about 1.7 to 1.

2.C. The actual cause of the neuralgic pain in Trother's syndrome is involvement of the mandibular nerve in the foramen ovale through which the tumor invades the calvarium.

3.A. Postherapetic neurlgia is a condition clinically similar to trigeminal neuralgia often occurs after attacks of herpes zoster of the fifth nerve.

4.C. The paratrigeminal syndrome is a disease characterized by severe headache or pain in the area of the trigeminal distribution with signs of ocular sympathetic paralysis.

5.C. In some patients the onset of the paroxysm occurs at exactly the same time of day and, for this reason, the disease has been referred to as "alam clock."

6.C. Horton's syndrome is caused by vasodilatation involving the internal maxillary artery, a branch of the external carotid, particularly that portion supplying the sphenopalatine region.

7.B. Also known as Cluster headache or Lower half headache.

8.D. Orolingual paresthesia is also caused by diabetes, psychogenic factors, trigeminal neuralgia, periodontal disease etc.

9.D. The auriculotemporal syndroma is an unusal phenomenon, which arises as a result of damage to the auriculotemporal nerve and subsequent reinnervation of sweat glands by parasympathetic salivary fibers.

10.A. Patients exhibit profuse lacrimation when food is eaten, particularly hot or spicy foods.

11.C. Seventh nerve paralysis is also known as Bell's palsy.

12.B. Recurrent attacks of facial paralysis, identical with Bell's palsy, associated with multiple episodes of non-pitting, non-inflammatory painless edema of the face, cheilitis granulomatosa, and fissured tongue is known as Melkerson-Rosenthal syndrome.

13.D. In glassopharyngeal neuralgia, patient usually has a trigger zone in the posterior oropharynx or tonsillar fossa.

14.D. These zones are difficult to localize but can be found by careful probing.

15.C. Facial and jaw weakness occurs in some patients.

16.A. Charcot's triad is a well known diagnostic triad characteristic of multiple sclerosis but not invariably present.

17.B. Multiple sclerosis is also known as disseminated sclerosis.

18.C. Multiple sclerosis is an acute or chronic, remittent or progressive disease of unknown etiology, but usually classified as one of the demyelinating disease affecting chiefly the white of the central nervous system.

19.A. Meniere's disease is characterized by deafness, tinnitus and vertigo.

20.D. The increased endolymphatic fluid pressure appears to diminish and distort the response to stimulation of the end organs of the labyrinth and cochlea.

21.A. Migraine is a syndrome presenting manifestation of diffuse disturbances in body function occurring during headache, irritability, and nausea.

22.C. Eagle's syndrome consists of either elongation of the styloid process or ossification of the stylohyoid ligament.

23.D. Eagle's syndrome is characterized by dysphagia, sore throat, otalgia, glossodynia, headache, vague orofacial pain etc.

24.D.

25.A. Ptosis is the drooping of the eyelid due to paresis of the smooth muscle elevator of the upper lid.

26.B. Also known as pterygoid Levator Synkinesis.

27.C. Hypertrophy is a secondary myopathy.

28.C. Myositis is a primary myopathy including dermatomyositis and myositis ossificans.

29.A. This disease is best described as a rapidly progressive muscle disease usually beginning in early childhood, presenting strong familial transmission with or without pseudo-hypertrophy.

30.B. But even the facial muscles may be involved.

31.D. CPK elevation occurs prior to the clinical manifestations of the disease in the males.

32.A. The lips develop a characteristic of looseness and protrusion, which have been described as tapir lips, a part of the myopathic facies, and the patient, is unable to the whistle or smile.

33.D. Mild restricted muscular dystrophy is a slowly progressive proximal myopathy, which primarily involves the muscle of the shoulder and face and has a weak familial incidence.

34.A. Myopathic facies is also known as swan neck.

35.B. Congenital myotonia is an anomaly of muscular contraction.

36.C. The degree of myotonia varies, but is generally severe and affects all sketetal muscles, especially those of the lower limbs.

37.A. The muscles are large, and patients with this disease are described as presenting a Herculean appearance.

38.B. Paramyotonia is manifested by cramping, stiffness and weakness of the muscles of the face and neck, fingers and hands upon exposure to cold.

39.B. Hypotonia is a reduction or complete absence of tonus in muscles.

40.D. Myasthenia gravis is a chronic disease characterized by progressive weakness of skeletal musceles, particularly those innervated by the cranial nerves.

41.C. Diplopia and ptosis, along with drooping of the face, lend a sorrowful appearance to the patient.

42.C. The messeteric atrophy produces a narrowing of the lower half of the face, which, the facial musculature, gives the patient a characteristic myopathic facies and swan neck.

43.D. Patients with this disease sometimes manifest a mild anemia or leukocytosis. In addition, creatinemia is a constant finding.

44.D. Entire groups of muscles become transformed into bone with resulting limitation of movement. The patient becomes transformed into a rigid organism sometimes encountered in circuses as the petrified man.

45.D. Horseback riders and jockeys develop Rider's bone in the thigh adductors.

46.A. Congenital facial diplegia is a nonfamilial deficient development of cranial muscles consisting of facial diplegia with bilaterial paralysis of the ocular muscles.

47.D. Congenital facial diplegia is usually manifested in infancy during the first dew days of life by failure to close the eyes during sleep.

48.D. Atrophy of muscle refers to a decrease in the size of individual muscle fibers which were once normal.

49.B. Hypertrophy of muscle refers to an increase in size of individual muscle fibers. This should be sepereated from pseudohypertrophy.

50.C. No cure for the disease is known, even though the pnognosis is good in the relapsing type.

19

Miscellaneous

All India PGDEE 2004

1. Thistle-tube appearance of pulp chamber is a feature of:

A. Coronal dentin dysplasia
B. Regional odontodysplasia
C. Dentinogenesis imperfecta
D. Amelogenesis imperfecta

2. Which of the following is not a feature of torus mandibularis?

A. Common in mongoloids
B. Present on the lingual surface of mandible above the mylohyoid line
C. Usually bilateral
D. May or may not associated with torus palatinus

3. Fordyce's (spots) granules in oral cavity arise from:

A. Mucous glands
B. Sebaceous glands
C. Taste buds
D. Minor salivary glands

4. The most common malignant tumor of adult males in India is:

A. Oropharyngeal carcinoma
B. Gastric carcinoma
C. Colo-rectal carcinoma
D. Lung cancer

5. The presence of higher amounts of proline-rich proteins (PRP) can have what kind of effect on caries causation?

A. Caries promoting since they help in bacterial

B. Make tooth surface resistant to caries since it enhance fluoride action

C. It has role during tooth mineralization only therefore no effect on caries

D. Aid in super saturation of saliva therefore make tooth resistant to caries

6. Among the common food items, fluoride is found in higher PPM in:

A. Pineapple
B. Tea
C. Sea fish
D. Coconut water

7. Fluoride is carried in the blood via:

A. Plasma
B. RBCs
C. Both Plasma and RBC
D. WBCs

8. Mulberry molars are characteristic features of:

A. Severe fluorosis

B. Trauma at the time of birth

C. Congenital syphilis

D. Due to chronic suppurative abscess in overlying gingival tissue

9. Famous Vipeholm study was conducted to:

A. To find out role of sticky and non-sticky form of sugars on dental caries

B. To find out the role of water fluoridation on dental caries

C. To find out role of xylitol on dental caries

D. All of the above

10. Etiology of mucocele is related to:

A. Mechanical trauma to the minor salivary gland excretory duct

B. Salivary calculi in the excretory duct major salivary gland

C. Acute infections

D. Smoking tobacco

11. **The main causative organism in Ludwigs angina is:**
    A. *Streptococcus viridans* B. *Staphylococcus albus*
    C. *Staphylococcus aureus* D. *Streptococcus haemolyticus*

12. **Which of the following terms refers to a type of fusion in which the formed teeth are joined only along the line of cementum:**
    A. Gemination B. Fusion
    C. Concrescence D. Dilaceration

13. **Which is a degeneration disorder characterized by atrophic changes of the deeper structures (e.g. fat, muscle, cartilage and bone) involving one side of the face:**
    A. Scleroderma B. Parry-Romberg syndrome
    C. Miescher's syndrome D. Peutz-Jeghers syndrome

14. **Virus responsible for infectious mononucleosis is:**
    A. RNA Paramyxo virus B. Varicella zoster virus
    C. Epstein-Barr virus D. Coxsackie virus A 16

15. **Name the lesions which is not a radiolucent lesion of the jaws:**
    A. Ameloblastoma
    B. Cherubism
    C. Focal periapical osteopetrosis
    D. Odontogenic cyst

16. **Name the lesion where cotton wool, multifocal radiodense conglomerates is not seen usually:**
    A. Gardner's syndrome B. Cemento-osseous dysplasia
    C. Paget's disease D. Fibrous dysplasia

17. **The syndrome of geographic tongue should be treated by:**
    A. Excision of the lesion
    B. Penicillin therapy
    C. Topical application of Nystatin
    D. Routine observation at recall time

18. The clinical picture of hairs in black hairy tongue is caused by hyperkeratinized hyperplastic:

A. Filiform papillae
B. Fungiform papillae
C. Vallate papillae
D. Filiform and fungiform papillae

All India PGDEE 2005

1. Ectodermal dysplasia is:

A. Autosomal recessive B. Autosomal dominant
C. X-linked dominant D. X-linked recessive

2. Enamel hypoplasis is not feature of:

A. Osteopetrosis
B. Down's syndrome
C. Some types of epidermolysis bullosa
D. Cleidocranial

3. Which of the following dentitions shows the highest frequency of occurrence of supernumerary teeth?

A. Maxillary deciduous dentition
B. Maxillary permanent dentition
C. Mandibular deciduous dentition
D. Mandibular permanent dentition

4. Hypercementosis of the entire dentition is a feature of:

A. Alber-Schonberg disease
B. Paget's disease
C. Lathyrism
D. Low grade periapical infammation

5. The permanent anterior tooth that most often shows variation in size is the:

A. Mandibular canine B. Mandibular central incisor
C. Maxillary canine D. Maxillary lateral incisor

6. **Which of the following teeth is most likely to be congenitally missing?**
   - A. Maxillary central incisor
   - B. Mandibular canine
   - C. Mandibular second premolar
   - D. Maxillary first premolar

7. **The term refers to a type of fusion in which the formed teeth are joined only along the line of cementum:**
   - A. Gemination
   - B. Fusion
   - C. Concrescence
   - D. Dilacerations

All India PGDEE 2006

1. **Which one of the following is the cause of dilacerations?**
   - A. Trauma to the tooth germ during root development.
   - B. Abnormal displacement of tooth germ during root development.
   - C. Abnormal proliferation of enamel epithelium during tooth development.
   - D. Abnormal displacement of ameloblasts during tooth formation.

2. **In the taurodontism, the teeth exhibit:**
   - A. Elongated, large pulp chambers and short roots
   - B. Elongated, small pulp chambers and short roots
   - C. Elongated, small pulp chambers and large roots
   - D. Short, small pulp chambers and large roots

3. ***Pemphigus vulgaris* is characterzed by:**
   - A. Acanthosis
   - B. Acantholysis
   - C. Auspilz's sign
   - D. Wickham's striae

4. **The important microorganism for dentinal caries is:**
   - A. *Actinomyosis actinobacillus*
   - B. *Borrelia vincentii*
   - C. *Streptococcus mutans*
   - D. *Streptococcus viridans*

5. **Which of the following is not responsible for endogenous**

staining of teeth during development?

A. Tetracycline B. Rh incompatibility
C. Neonatal liver disease D. Vitamin C deficiency

6. A polyp may arise in connection with:

A. Chronic open pulpitis B. Pulp necrosis
C. Acute pulpitis D. A chronic periapical lesion

7. Blue sclera is characteristic of:

A. Amelogenesis imperfecta
B. Tetracycline hypoplasia
C. Fluorosis
D. Osteogenesis imperfecta

8. Which of the following is the diagnostic characteristic of peripheral giant cell granuloma?

A. Mass of granulation tissue
B. Multinuclear giant cells
C. Keliod like enlargement
D. Epithelium is atrophic in some areas

9. Dense in dente is most commonly seen in:

A. Premolars B. Paramolars
C. Lateral incisors D. Maxillary canine

10. Taurodontism is usually seen in:

A. Mesiodens B. Incisor with talon/cusp
C. Mandibular first molar D. Maxillary premolars

11. Which of the following conditions is least likely to present as an eccentric osteolytic lesion:

A. Aneurysmal bone cyst B. Giant cell tumor
C. Fibrous cortical defect D. Simple bone cyst

12. Acinic cell carcinomas of the salivary gland arise most often in the:

A. Parotid salivary gland
B. Minor salivary glands
C. Submandibular salivary gland
D. Sublingual salivary gland

13. Mixed tumors of the salivary glands are:

A. Most common in submandibular gland
B. Usually malignant
C. Most common in parotid gland
D. Associated with calculi

Explanations

All India PGDEE 2004

1.A. In coronal dentin dysplasia, permanent teeth exhibit an abnormally large pulp chamber in the coronal portion of the tooth, often described as "thistte tube"in shape.

2.D. This growth on the lingual surface of the mandible occurs above the mylohyoid line, usually opposite the bicuspid teeth.

3.B. Fordyce's granules appear as small yellow spots, either discretely separated or forming relatively large plaques, often projecting slightly above the surface of the tissue.

4.A. Due to tobacco chewing habit in adult males oropharyngeal carcinoma is most common malignant tumor.

5.C. PRP has effect only on tooth mineralization and no direct effect on carious process.

6.C. In general, the leaves of plants contain more fluoride than the stems, and the skin of fruit contains more than the pulp.

7.C. Fluoride is carried in the blood via plasma and red blood cells.

8.C. Mulberry molars are also known as moon's molars or Fournier's molars.

9.A. Vipeholm study concluded that sticky sugars are more cariogenic.

10.A. Mucocele is also known as mucous retention cyst.

11.D. Most cases of Ludwig's angina are a mixed infection, but streptococci are almost invariably present.

12.C. Conerescence arise as a result of traumatic injury or crowding of teeth with resorption of the interdental bone so that the two roots are in approximate contact and become fused by the deposition of cementum between them.

13.B. Scleroderma is characterized by progressive fibrosis of skin and multiple organs and by vascular insufficiency through abnormalities in arterioles and capillaries.

14.C. Infections mononucleosis is also known as kissing disease.

15.C. The density of the bone is such that the roots of the teeth are nearly invisible on the dental reoentgenograms.

16.A. Gardner's syndrome consists of (i) multiple polyposis of the large intestine, (ii) osteomas, (iii) multiple epidermoid or sebaceous cysts (iv) desmoid tumors (v) impacted supernumerany and permanent teeth.

17.D. Since the etiology is unknown, the treatment is empirical.

18.A. Hairy tongue is characterized by hypertrophy of fillform papillae of tongue, with lack of normal desquamation, which may be extensive and form a thick matted layer on the dorsal surface.

All India PGDEE 2005

1.D. Hereditory ectodermal dysplasia is a syndrome characterized by congenital dysplasia of one or more ectodermal structures. Its common manifestations are hypohidrosis, hypotrichosis and hypodontia. In majority of cases it shows x-linked recessive character.

2.C. Enamel hypoplasia is present in epidermolysis bullosa dystrophic recessive while absent in epidermolysis bullosa dystrophic dominant and in epidermolysis cullosa simple.

3.B. Superneumary teeth are more common in permanent teeth than in deciduous dentition. Approximately 90% of all supernumary teeth occur in maxilla. The most common supernumary tooth is mesiodens, which is situated between the maxillary central incisors.

4.B. Hypercementosis is regressive change of teeth characterized by the excessive amount of secondary cementum on root surface. Hypercementosis is a common feature of Paget's disease.

5.D. Variation in the size of tooth is manifested as microdontia and macrodontia. Macrodontia is relatively uncommon.

Microdontia of a single tooth is a common condition. It affects most often the maxillary lateral incisor among anterior teeth and the third molar among posterior teeth.

6.C. Studies on the frequency of missing teeth shows that third molar are most often congenitally missing permanent teeth followed by second premolars.

7.C. Concrescence is actually a type of fusion, which takes place after root has been completely formed. Here the teeth are united by cementum only. It arises as a result of traumatic injury or crowding of teeth.

All India PGDEE 2006

1.A. Dilaceration is sharp bend or curve in the root or crown of a formed tooth. It is due to trauma during the period in which the tooth is forming.

2.A. In taurodontism the body of the tooth is enlarged at the expense of the roots. The tooth involved are mostly permanent molars. The pulp chamber of involved tooth is much greater in apico-occlusal height than normal and the roots area short.

3.B. Pemphigus is a chronic skin disease characterized by the appearance of vesicles, bullae, and fluid filled blisters that develop in cycle. Pemphigus vulgaris is most common form of pemphigus. In pemphigus vesicle or bulla is intraepithelial, thus weakens the intacellular bridge resulting in acantholysis.

4.C. Microorganism for dentinal caries is *Streptococcus mutans.*

5.D. Those stain, which are incorporated into tooth structure are intrinsic stain. These develop due to tetracycline therepy, erythroblastosis fetalis and in porphyria. Vitamin C deficiency leads to bleeding gums of scurvy.

6.A. Pulp polyp is chromic hyperplastic pulpitis. It shows exuberant proliferation of infammed dental pulp tissue. It occurs almost exclusively in children and young adult and involves teeth with large open carious lesions.

7.D. Osteogenesis imperfecta is also called as brittle bone disease because its chief characteristic is extreme fragility and porosity of bone with proneness to fracture. The second characteristic of it is the occurrence of pale blue sclera.

8.B. Peripheral giant cell granuloma also called giant cell epulis. It histologically shows nonencapsulated mass of tissue composed of delicate reticular and fibrillar connective tissue stroma containing large number of young spindle shaped connective tissue cells and multinucleated giant cells.

9.C. Dense in dente is a developmental anomaly that occurs due to an invagination in the surface of tooth before its calcification is completed. Permanent maxillary lateral incisors are commonly affected by this defect.

10.C. Taurodontism is a condition in which the pulp chamber is elongated, enlarged and extands in the roots

11.D. In simple bone cyst failure of organization of blood clot occurs and subsequent degeneration of clot produce empty cavity with in the bone. The lesion increases in size due to restriction of venous drainage and ceases when the lesion reaches the cortical layer of bone. Thus, bone expansion is not a common finding in simple bone cyst.

12.A. Acinic cell carcinoma is also called serous cell adenoma. It resembles pleomorphic adenoma in gross appearance. This tumor occurs chiefly in the parotid salivary gland.

13.C. Mixed tumors of the salivary glands are called pleomorphic adenoma. It is benign in nature. Most commonly pleomorphic adenoma involves the parotid gland by 90% of all the major salivary gland.